TABLE OF CONTENTS

Breast Care

Bronchitis

Bruises

Bursitis

Burns

Cancer / Tumors

Chicken Pox

Choking

Childbirth

Circulation

Cleansing (Colon)

Colic

Colds

Colitis

Constipation

Corns

Cough

Cradle Cap

Cramps

Croup

Dandruff

Dermatitis

Diabetes

Diaper Rash

Diarrhea

Dislocations

Dizziness

Dry Skin

Ear Infections / Aches

Eczema

Emphysema

Energy

Eye Care

Facial Care

Fever

Fingernails

Foot Care

Frostbite

Gas

Gout

Hair Care / Loss

Headaches

Heartburn

Heart Care

Hemorrhoids

Hepatitis

Hernia / Rupture

Hearing Problems

Herpes Simplex

Hiccups

Hives

Hoarseness / Laryngitis

Hyperactivity

Hypoglycemia

Indigestion

Inflammation

Insomnia

Itching

Lactation

Leg Pains

Liver Care

Lumbago

Lungs

Lupus

Lymph Glands

Measles

Memory

Menopause / Hot Flashes

Menstruation

Migraines

Miscarriage

Morning Sickness

Motion Sickness

Mouth Sores

Mucus / Congestion

Mumps

Nausea

Nerves

Nightmares

Nosebleed

Osteoporosis

Pain

Parasites

Pet Care

Phlebitis

Pituitary

Pleurisy

Poison Ivy

Poisoning

Polyps

Pregnancy Tips

Prickly Heat

Prostate Gland

Psoriasis

Rashes

Rheumatism

Scarlet Fever

Scars

Senility

Shingles

Shock

Skin Cracks

Meet the Author

The Complete Health System

No Sceince Can Extend Your Life But We Can Offer a Better Quality of Life

©Copyright 2012 by Dr. Harry Jay

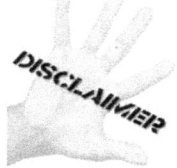

DISCLAIMER AND TERMS OF USE AGREEMENT:

(Please Read This Before Using This Book)

Introduction - Economy Squeezes the American Dream

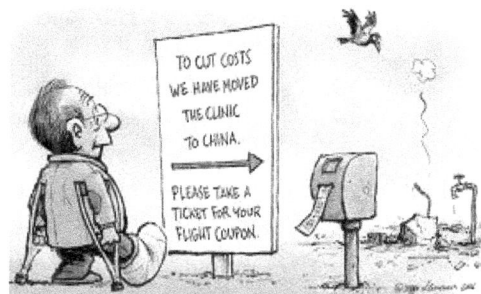

I read an article the other day titled..."Economy Squeezes the American Dream". It talked about the current economy's effect on the "American Dream." From the very first sentence, I knew that the writer knew NOTHING about what the American dream was. The very first sentence of the article was..."Work hard, play by the rules and tomorrow will be better than today." AMAZING!

Are you kidding me, I thought? The "work hard" part I got. It's a necessity to be able to live your dream lifestyle no matter where you live. But, "play by the rules and tomorrow will be better than today." Excuse me, but that is pure unadulterated garbage! Here is what happens when you play by the rules....

1. You go to college and spend a ridiculous amount of money on a degree you in most cases will never use or need.

2. You get a job that pays you little, but forces you to work 50 to 70 hours per week to make ends meet.

3. You most likely have no job security and a boss and employer that cares little about you.

4. You get the "privilege" of taking one vacation a year if you are lucky.

5. You work until you are at least 65 and possibly longer so that you can have just enough money to live out the rest of your days. Plus you no longer get a gold watch and you are lucky to get a pat on your head and a thank you.

Sound like the "American Dream" to you? Sounds more like a nightmare to me. If you "play by the rules," that is a pretty likely scenario for you! Truth is, the article may have had good intentions, but was WAY off. Those that have been able to live the "American Dream," or to live their dream lifestyle no matter where they are from, have never played by the rules.

Yes, hard work has always been a required element to living out your dream lifestyle. But those that have dream lifestyles almost always create their own rules. They are what's called "self-made."

In fact, of the 15 wealthiest people in the world as of 2008, 10 of them are self made and 5 of them inherited the money. Of the 10 that are self made billionaires, a whopping 9 are high school or college dropouts!

Am I preaching against getting an education? No; but if you want to live your dream lifestyle, you have to take charge of your own life. You have to make your own rules. And, you have to make things happen for yourself.

Many years ago, after being let go from my job 3 weeks before Christmas with a baby on the way and by an employer who cared little about me or my family no matter how hard I worked, I took charge of my life.

Today... I work when I want to. I play when I want to. I vacation when I want to. I can afford the things that I want. I am my own boss!

And....I definitely DO NOT play by the rules. I make my own.

If you want to play by the rules, go ahead. But, don't expect any sort of dream lifestyle out of it. If you want to start taking control of your life...If you want to enjoy life as it was meant to be enjoyed...If you want to be free from the prison that is the 9 to 5 world...If you want to take control instead of being controlled...YOU have to make it happen! Start making it happen today. I will show you how now by taking control of your health.

"The human mind will first seek to alleviate pain before it seeks pleasure"

The Clown

In New York City, on a bright spring day, a man dodges the crowds of pedestrians as he makes his way to a downtown Manhattan skyscraper. Anyone who would look would see the man was burdened; his hunched shoulders, the look of sadness in his face and eyes, betrayed the man's inner gloom. The man soon arrives at his destination, an appointment made months in advance, with one of New York's leading psychiatrists. The man is ushered into the doctor's plush office, and sits heavily in the offered chair.

The doctor asks in a quiet manner, "What seems to be the problem?"

The man hesitates at first, and then finds his voice. He clears his throat and almost whispers, "I really don't know, doctor. I haven't smiled in years. I have no joy in my life. And worst of all, I have no idea why?"

The doctor nods his head, in understanding, and then proceeds to administer a comprehensive battery of tests, beginning with a physical, to determine the cause of the man's problem. Afterwards, in a private session, the doctor counsels, "I find nothing wrong with you, sir," he begins with a sigh, "but I want you to try something. There is a circus in town this week. They say it is the finest circus in the world. There is a clown with this circus with a reputation of making everyone laugh. I want you to go and see this clown. Possibly, he can restore your joy."

The man looks up from wringing his hands. And with tears in his eyes, he stares at the doctor. Almost in a choking voice the man says, "Doctor, I am that clown!"

On the outside, the man was the epitome of joy... a clown, but on the inside, he was a barren and lonely man. How many people do you know do the same thing? It is human nature to project what you want the world to see *(we call this reputation or a facade),* and behind close doors, the real you comes out *(we call this character).* Remember, a facade is just a mask!

We are what we are in the dark; all the rest is reputation. What God looks at is what we are in the dark-the imaginations of our minds; the thoughts of our heart; the habits of our bodies, these are the things that mark us in God's sight.
- Oswald Chambers –

Nutrition and fitness represent one of the largest industries on the net today. But with all the pertinent information and products available, the only thing they can do and do well is increase the quality of your life rather than the quantity of your life. Since it is true our days are numbered, it makes sense that these days should be filled with meaning, and a peaceful existence designed to maximize the "quality" of life. But another human trait has a way of consistently rearing its ugly head: "People are more interested in relief versus cure!" As long as there is no pain and they look good, people seem content to operate and live their lives within this facade. This too is wrong and pardon my pun but it is also "dead' wrong! Always go for QUALITY! The quantity of your life will take care of yourself.

Toxins and Toxaemia

The human body is finely designed to stay in balance (homeostasis) in terms of tissue building up (called anabolism). and tissue breaking down (called catabolism). An excess of one over the other, is called a metabolic imbalance. Toxaemia (the build up of toxins in the body), first occurs as a process of metabolism. Old cells are constantly being replaced by new cells. In fact three hundred billion or more old cells are called toxic, and must be removed, as soon as possible, by the immune system, through one of four channels of elimination: bowels, bladder, lungs, and skin...and sometimes hurling.

The problem of Toxaemia first occurs when your body is not eliminating toxics at the same rate the toxics are being reproduced.

The second way Toxaemia occurs is from the by-products of foods that are not properly digested. The major portions of the foods we eat are processed. Because most of our food has been altered from its original state and we are not biologically adapted to deal with this altered food, the by-products of the incomplete digestion form a certain amount of residue, which builds up in the body. This residue is also called Toxic. Regarding your body weight, common sense will tell you that if more of this toxic weight is built up, rather than eliminated, then obesity will occur.

TOXAEMIA IS THE NUMBER 1 CAUSE OF OBESITY AND NOT A HIGH CALORIE DIET!!! An excess of body fat holds the toxic wastes and attempts to keep the toxins away from the organs of the body.

Here is one of the best diets I have seen on the market today that addresses toxaemia: Toxins are acidic by nature, hence the body retains water to dilute and neutralize the acids in the toxins, adding even more weight and bloatedness. If the problem goes unchecked, the ultimate result is not only obesity, but also general discomfort, lethargy and a DISRUPTION OF THE ENERGY FLOW OF THE BODY! In fact, a good deal of the body's finite energy supply is used to eliminate the toxins in the body.

Cleansing of the system frees up energy.

The following problems occur directly because of Toxaemia: cellulite, irritable bowel syndrome, arthritis, swollen ankles/joints, bad breath, slow metabolism (increase in weight), ulcers, digestive problems, migraines, bad skin, weak hair and nails, low immune system, and kidney problems.

Something to think about...

The concept of total optimum health is not new. This term has been bantered about the healthcare field for years. What is unique however, and rather innovative about the "Fit-4-Life" Complete Health System, is my belief that total optimum health is only achieved when the needs of the body, mind, soul, and spirit, as they interrelate with one another, are met or exceeded.

In other words, the mind affects the body and the body affects the mind!

There is a common belief among leading social scientists that intellect and emotion never meet. In other words, they are mutually exclusive, and never interrelate with each other in our decision-making processes. Can this be true? Let me give an example, and then you can decide. When a person sees a baby crying, the action required to pick-up that baby (intellect), has no bearing whatsoever on the need to pick-up that baby (emotion). In other words, what is required to raise that baby off the floor against the law of gravity has nothing to do with the desire to hold the baby and give it love and a nurturing environment. Yes, a physical action is quite different from a nurturing action but the point I am making is that they are both ACTIONS; hence, they are interrelated. **Why is this so important? By understanding the body's relationships, a person can acquire a better quality of life. No science can extend your life, but science can and does offer a better quality of life.**

My beliefs regarding health goes against the grain of accepted health field thought. Contrary to popular belief, most people believe that systematic science puts forth a theory and when this theory is proven then it becomes a law of science. Einstein put for the theory of relativity in 1903 (e=mc^2) and it became the Law of Relativity in 1933 not because anybody proved it. This IS NOT what systemic science does at all! A theory becomes a law if we CANNOT DISPROVE THE THEORY WRONG. This is called "falsification" and this is how systematic science operates. What you are about to read will be an adventure in thought and practice. The health world has been telling you for decades to limit your protein and fat intake, and to eat a high-carbohydrate diet. It is our contention that this high carbohydrate/low fat diet is causing major problems with the health and well being of many Americans. The incidence of heart disease, diabetes, and cancer are on the rise. So what has caused these problems?

This book will discuss these topics plus much more. Later in the book, we will also discuss the latest in food and health technology…the cutting edge of nutritional research. We will also discuss the need for supplements. Do you really need to take all those pills? Walking into a health store can be a mind-boggling experience. Even most professional health people are hard pressed to tell you how to choose a good supplement. Also, I want you to pay extra close attention to the chapters dealing with HGH and the Glycemic Food Index. These are very important chapters, on weight maintenance and body science. For you ladies, we have included some interesting reports on problems that affect the female body. In my book "Applied Mind Science," I delve into how the mind affects the body not only in regards to health but also in the total quality of life. I strongly recommend you read this book! It is well worth the effort and cost and you can find it on Amazon.com. Last, I am going to reveal some extremely interesting research form my Applied Mind Sciences research unit regarding energy psychology as well as energy neutraceuticals. So, please read on and learn some very interesting facts. Ignorance need not be a science!

The sciences and how they interrelate

Let's begin by laying down a solid foundation just to keep things in perspective. As previously said, every human being is made up of mind, body, soul, and spirit. The health of a human being centers on all four of these characteristics. A physical disease will affect mental health, and a mental disease will affect physical health.

It is important to understand that all medical science and practices come from a religious foundation. From the 5th century B. C. up until the mid-1800s, all medicine was practiced based on humoralistic beliefs and techniques. This practice is attributed to the Greek physician, Hippocrates, but holds a significant resemblance to, the ancient Hindu system called the, "Ayurvedic" system. Humors are the fluids in the human body. This was the reason a person was "bled," and leeches employed, to remove excess fluids. Once this quackery was debunked, western medicine turned to allopathic practice, or "Allopathy."

Allopathy is a method of treating disease with remedies that produce effects different (dissimilar) from those caused by the disease itself. Allopathy is the system of medicine practiced today by medical doctors (M.D.s) and relies solely on scientific experimentation. Allopathy differs from naturopathy; insofar, as the former practices curative medicine, and the latter practices preventative medicine. Allopathic medicine uses medications and surgery. Naturopathic physicians employ, natural, or alternative methods.

Homeopathy is a system of medicine, or method of treating disease, with remedies that produce effects similar to those caused by the disease itself.

Osteopathy and Chiropractic systems are methods using manipulation of the skeleton, to cure problematic parts of the body. None of the methods used today, regard the "mind" as influencing the healing process. This is very sad.

Psychology was born in the mid-1800s too. It used to be called philosophy but the desire to make it a "science' overcame the logic of what it truly is and today it operates under a blanket of respectability that is unwarranted.

Remember, systematic science first proposes a theory and when it cannot be disproved (falsification) the theory then becomes a law. All of psychology is based on the mechanism of the mind: belief systems + thought = behavior/conduct. Then in 1957, a noted psychologist name Leon Festinger proposed the theory of "cognitive dissonance," which states that actions are inconsistent with beliefs. This one theory completely contradicts all of psychology! In psychology's almost 150 years of existence, not one theory has ever been proven or disproven.

THERE ARE NO LAWS OF PSYCHOLOGY...not one! None of psychology's methods used today regard the "mind" as influencing the healing process.

To better understand, the human being, as it relates to others as well as its environment, I need you to thoroughly understand the concept that the "Complete Person" is made up of mind, body, soul, and spirit. Physiologically speaking, the body operates around the central nervous system; made up of two sub-systems called the somatic nervous system (this is the system that gives you volitional control of your muscles and skeletal movements) and the autonomic nervous system (this is the system, which regulates our glands and correlates with our emotions). The central nervous system includes the brain, and spinal cord. The autonomic nervous system tells the brain, which stimuli have been received; the brain responds based upon how it has been programmed. Since an individual is the sum total of his/her experiences, the brain is programmed based on these experiences, as well as perceived experience. The brain IS NOT the mind! The mind resides in the brain but they are two separate and distinct entities. The best way to describe all of the "parts," using computer terminology, is the autonomic nervous system is the software, the brain is the hardware, and the mind is the hard drive. You must never forget the "Complete Person" concept, as you attempt to practice proper health protocols. Every book has a system, a diet, a proven way to lose weight...the claims touted are amazing.

DON'T BELIEVE ANY OF IT!

☆ If you have a strong desire to be healthy, simply eat good wholesome food; stay away from processed food and adulterated fats.

☆ Eat natural things like nuts, fruits, and vegetables.

☆ Remember, too: eat in moderation and only when you are hungry. BALANCE is what you should seek!

☆ As for supplements, they are not food. They are meant to supplement a diet.

To begin to understand your body, you must first understand the relationships your body employs, as it strives for optimum health. As a behavioral scientist trained in both secular and non-secular protocols, I have noticed that the secular side of the equation tends to view illness of the body, or the mind, completely separate from the soul and spirit. I referred to this briefly at the end of my book "Addictions":

Secular psychologists believe that the cause of illness is because of the way we **choose** to think or believe. Using cognitive therapy (having a basis in or reducible to empirical factual knowledge.), they attempt to change a person's behavior and feelings. But, we now know that illness is cured **not by changing our feelings or behavior**, but **by changing our beliefs and thoughts**. Does this sound like double-speak to you? One of the things we will discuss is how men/women constantly confuse similar sounding terms, which have very separate and distinct meanings. In the following, men/women commonly confuse:

☆ **Faith vs. Hope**

☆ **Righteousness vs. Goodness**

☆ **Freedom vs. Liberty**

- ☆ **Rules vs. Ethics**
- ☆ **Quality vs. Quantity**
- ☆ **Quality of Life vs. Standard of Living**
- ☆ **Love vs. Lust**
- ☆ **Obligation vs. Legalism**
- ☆ **Wealth vs. Money**
- ☆ **Want vs. Need**
- ☆ **Machismo vs. Manhood**
- ☆ **Femininity vs. Womanhood**
- ☆ **War vs. Conflict**
- ☆ **Well-being vs. Being well**
- ☆ **Cause vs. Effect**
- ☆ **Relief vs. Cure**
- ☆ **Rationalization vs. Right**
- ☆ **Promise vs. Oath (Vow)**
- ☆ **Discipline vs. Punishment**
- ☆ **Taste vs. Substance**
- ☆ **Pain vs. Suffering**
- ☆ **Self-Control vs. Willpower**

Can you honestly tell me the difference between liberty and freedom? Cause and effect, is one example of this problem. Using my statement above, beliefs (belief systems) and thoughts, CAUSE our behavior and feelings, which are in turn, the effects of both belief and thought. In order to change your behavior and feelings, you must first change the cause; which are your belief systems. You need to reread this paragraph again slowly, because it is very important. Belief Systems evoke thoughts, which evoke actions, which equal behavior and feelings.

Many people have mental illnesses, which manifests itself in psychosomatic (self-caused) symptoms of depression, anxiety, chronic fatigue, drug addiction, insomnia, ulcers etc. The mind truly does affect the body! Think of someone who has wronged you in the past, and see how your body responds. You become anxious and stressed. You begin to think of revenge, as your heart races, and your ears pound. Adrenaline begins to course through your body. You cannot separate the two entities (body and mind always interact), even though there are some occult religions that claim to free you from your body by meditation and visualization. In the above example, you react the way you do based on how your mind has been programmed. This is your character. A child reared in a family, which uses violence to solve problems, uses violence in its own life, to solve problems, because this is how the child was programmed.

A lifestyle is made up of various habits. All people respond, to various stimuli, based on how they are trained. Over the years, people have learned to react to certain situations with a predictable behavioral pattern. Habits through practice turn into behavior - both good and bad. Like I said, not all habits are good habits either. A person suffers from his/her own personal problems, like you, and the stress and anxiety his/her choices bring. Wrongful choices evoke stress and anxiety. This is important to understand completely. Wrongful choices evoke suffering. This suffering takes the form of anxiety, stress, and the list of other psychosomatic ailments I previously listed. Here is a direct quote from one of my associates, psychologist Hobart Mowrer, that I think you will find quite interesting:

"Human anxiety is a result of dammed-up moral force rather than dammed-up libido. As this force seeps out into a man's consciousness (from his subconscious mind), **he experiences it not as guilt about a real fault or sin** (perception) **but as great anxiety. Anxiety is not the result of too little indulgence, but of too much, not of over-restraint and inhibition, but of irresponsibility, guilt, and immaturity. Above all, the eternal accomplishment of untold past generations, as imbedded in the conscience of modern men and women, is not a stupid, malevolent, archaic incubus** (evil spirit), **but a challenge and guide for the individual, in his quest for self-fulfillment and harmonious integration."**

Freud regarded anxiety as foreign, unfriendly, and destructive. However, Mowrer believes that conscience, and the anxiety it produces, can be transformed into guilt and moral fear, for which unhappy man can make some realistic adjustment. Mowrer's prescription: A changed attitude (belief system) toward social authority and its internal representative anxiety. We will also talk more about authority in just a little while.

"If a man's attitude is not changed, he will continue to seek relief from anxiety in such futile devices as tobacco, alcohol, gambling, sexual perversion, and gluttony."

Do you get it? Some of the things you do are caused by stress and anxiety, which have been caused by wrongful choices. Smoking, over-eating, drinking, and gambling, are just a few examples of the manifested behavior caused by stress and anxiety, which in turn, are caused by wrongful choices. These types of manifested behaviors act as a relief valve and defense mechanism. It follows that since wrongful choices are the true culprit to a life of bondage, to the effects of wrongful choices, then we need to learn how to develop correct choices. Let me take it one step further. People do not appear to see the difference between the matter part of an organism and the life part, which animates it. They seem to think that the organism itself is life. We all seem to suffer a similar problem of understanding. To put it in perspective, people do not appear to see the difference between their outward habits and the inward part that animates it. It is not their outward appearance that defines their habits but their inward experiences and anxieties, and this is where their habits are born. In other words, life is not your physical body. Life is what animates the body. Life is your spirit, but the soul of man has usurped the spirit's position and psychology is now forced to define "how" we live our lives based on the animating force of the soul instead of the spirit.

To summarize, the body contains the brain, which contains the mind, which contains the conscious and subconscious parts of the mind. The subconscious mind is made up of the desires, emotions and will or what I refer to as "DEW". This is where we get our feelings, attitudes, sentiments and opinions. This is where our dreams are born and failures grieved. This is the place where intricate processes are put into motion and life's decisions are contemplated. Here we find the conflicting emotions of love/hate, like/dislike, and attraction/repulsion. Here is our daily existence. It is the pollution of the subconscious mind that causes our problems. All manifested behavior stems from the subconscious mind! The soul of man is a term to describe this subconscious aspect of man. The ancient Hebrews defined the soul in two ways. They called the souls of animals "nefesh," which were souls that did not share the eternality nature of God, and the soul of man was called "neshama," which did share the eternality of God. All animals possess souls (science uses the term "breath" to describe the physical manifestation of the soul); it is our spirits, which makes us different. The mind is very important because this is the playground of poor choices. It is in the mind where all thought is first contemplated and it is in the mind where all action begins.

"On the inside, we are defined by what we lack, on the outside, what defines us is what we have."

What we lack on the inside is Truth and what we have on the outside is what the world uses to evaluate our success. Now getting back to the mind, we know that our minds can be used against us. Everyone has heard of brainwashing, mind-control, magic, hypnosis, etc. To live in the mind, we live as "consuming entities." We desire to take and not give back. Look around you, the world always wants more. We even call ourselves "consumers". The products we consume are offered up in the most appealing advertisements. They are "beautiful" and we want them. In olden times, our eyes were never bigger than our pocketbook. We didn't have credit cards back then. Today, we can consume on credit and this has led many into a life of financial subjugation.

"If you live as a consuming entity, you will always lose."

In other words, to get, you must give-you must sacrifice! Have you ever wondered why you have so many anxieties, phobias, worries and fears? Remember what I taught you above. The reality of this world is evil. So what is reality? I will tell you. This is reality:

"Life without war is impossible either in nature or in grace. The basis of physical, mental, moral and spiritual life is antagonism. Health is the balance between physical life and external nature, and it is maintained only by sufficient vitality on the inside against things on the outside.

Everything outside my physical life is designed to put me to death.

Things, which keep me going when I am alive, disintegrate me when I am dead. If I have enough fighting power, I produce the balance of health. The same is true of mental life. If I want to maintain a vigorous mental life, I have to fight, and in that way the mental balance called thought is produced. Morally it is the same. Everything that does not partake of the nature of virtue is the enemy of virtue in me, and it depends on what moral caliber I have whether I overcome and produce virtue (GOOD CHARACTER). Immediately I fight, I am moral in that particular. No man is virtuous because he cannot help it; virtue (character) is acquired.

Chapter 1: Do You Really Need All Those Supplements?

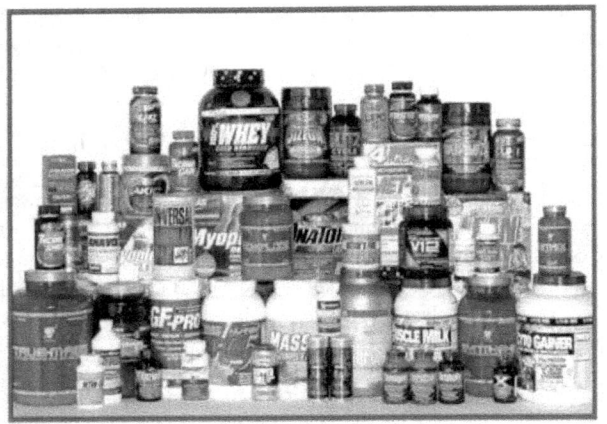

   In answering a question as complicated and important as this one, we must look to scientific fact rather than the host of opinions that bombard the American consumer. One fact is this: the optimum daily amounts of vitamins and minerals are far larger than the amounts that can be obtained in food. This is because of present day farming techniques and an increase in the amount of processed food Americans ingest daily. The quality has decreased and Americans have increased the quantity of consumption. Poor food and poor eating habits require us to use supplements.

Choosing a Responsibly Made Vitamin

   Vitamins either enable biochemical reactions in the body to take place more effectively, or they prevent specific substances from interfering with the biochemical reactions. **Why do I need to take vitamins?** If our soil was not depleted and we did not use pesticides and herbicides on our crops, which greatly reduce the bioavailability of the nutrients to be metabolized, and we ate fruits and vegetables within 6-days of harvesting, and we didn't heat process our food, and add preservatives to them-we wouldn't need to take vitamins. **What should I look for in a vitamin?** Consumers need to be well informed when making the decision to ingest any substance. In considering a supplement, the guidelines for determining if a supplement is responsibly made should include: Heat Processing and Tableting, Iron -Why it should NOT be present, Vitamin-C, Vitamin-D, Beta Carotene, B-Complexes, Chelation and Minerals, Timed-Released, and Synergists.

Heat Processing and Tableting

Look for a supplement that is not heat processed. Tablets are heat processed and capsules are not. Capsules cost the manufacturer more, so most manufacturers tend to use the tableting method. Capsules or pure powders deliver the highest potency. Also, fillers and binders are used to make a tablet hold together, and these binders may cause allergic reactions in some people. Many people think they are allergic to vitamins when they are really only allergic to the binder or filler. Also, tableting may cause extrusion of oil-soluble vitamins from the formulation. For example, a tablet press compresses at 5000 psi which can release beadleted oil-soluble Vitamin A from the protective coat. The Vitamin A then degrades rapidly.

Iron – Why it Should NOT be Present

Look for a complete vitamin/mineral supplement that does not contain iron. Studies have shown that "increased body iron stores are associated with an increase risk of cancer": New England Journal of Medicine. This does not refer to iron found in food or the iron found in protein powders, but to supplemental iron. Also, studies indicate that two-in-four hundred Caucasians have Hemochromatosis; an inherited disorder that causes iron overload and the symptoms can be quite severe. Iron deficiencies in males are rare. Some women do have iron deficiencies in which case an increase in dietary intake of iron rich foods may eliminate the problem. If dietary readjustment does not alleviate the deficiency, an iron supplement may be taken once or twice a week until serum iron levels reach the normal range.

Vitamin-C

The data on Vitamin-C is so extensive that it is unnecessary to validate its value. I would not take more than 500 mgs of Vitamin-C per day. **Megadoses are not advisable** (Are we really meant to consume 20-30 oranges a day? Does this make sense to you?). Megadoses of Vitamin-C depress sperm motility and decreases fertility. It also blunts the beneficial effects of chemotherapy treatment for breast cancer. Cancer cells have numerous receptors for Vitamin-C making it act as a growth tonic for cancer cells. Also, its own synergist, the bioflavonoids, should always accompany Vitamin-C. Vitamin-C does not occur in nature without its sisters, rutin and hesperidin-both bioflavonoids, and any well-made vitamin should mimic nature as closely as possible. Note: Smoking depletes almost 50% of the vitamin-C in the body.

Vitamin-D

Vitamin-D is a vitamin, which acts like a hormone and is the only vitamin the human body can manufacture. In its absence, calcium and phosphorus become immobile and leeching of these two minerals becomes inevitable. In addition, as we age, our ability to synthesize Vitamin-D slows to one-half. Though we need Vitamin-D, it is potentially very toxic, so a safe supplement will not contain large amounts of Vitamin-D. We do not recommend taking a Vitamin-D supplement. **If your body is getting the proper amount of essential fatty acids (Omega 3, 6, 9 oils) your body will make a sufficient amount of Vitamin-D.** Most of the Vitamin-D utilized in the body comes from sunlight interacting with the essential fatty acids in the skin. Therefore, supplemental Vitamin-D without the benefit of sunlight is insufficient for total health. Sun exposure (with sunscreen) should include 20-minutes of summer sun exposure and 40-minutes of winter sun exposure. Be advised that an excessive amount of Vitamin-D causes a magnesium deficiency in the body. Furthermore, megadoses of Vitamin-D irritate the lining of blood vessels and are one of the causes of atherosclerosis.

Beta Carotene

Beta Carotene (Pro-Vitamin A or plant derived Vitamin A) is a natural substance found in fruits and vegetables, which, once inside the body, converts to Vitamin A. Vitamin A is crucial in normal cellular control. Since the body must get Vitamin A from outside sources, when the body does not receive an adequate supply of Vitamin A, cell function becomes abnormal, and cell maturation does not take place. Cells deprived of Vitamin A dedifferentiate, and enter a state paralleling cancerous cells. Stress (including both colds and flu) can deplete up to 60% of the Vitamin A in the body. At St. Luke's Medical Center in Chicago, an important study involving beta-carotene and lung cancer was conducted. It involved 2,107 workers at the Western Electric Company in Chicago. Thirty-Three (33) of the men developed lung cancer, all related to cigarette smoking. The rate of cancer was lowest in those people consuming the highest amounts of beta-carotene foods and the highest in the group consuming the least amounts of beta-carotene foods. The actual ratio turned out to be an 8-to-1 difference in risk between the lowest and highest groups. Beta Carotene can actually negate gene mutation, which occurs when the body is exposed to environmental toxins such as cigarette smoke. The incidence of lung cancer in smokers (2 packs a day for 30-years) who consumed diets high in beta-carotene was similar to the incidence of lung cancer in non-smokers. This is phenomenal data evidencing the powerful anti-carcinogenic properties of beta-carotene. Unused Vitamin A is stored in the liver and can be toxic when taken for extended periods at high doses, where as beta-carotene is considered nontoxic at very high doses. A combination of beta-carotene and Vitamin A (in moderate doses) in a supplement is preferable.

B-Complexes

The B-Vitamins include: B-1 (Thiamin), B-2 (Riboflavin), B-5 (pantothenic acid), B-6 (pyridoxine), B-12 (Cobalamin), PABA (para-aminobenzoic acid), folate (folic acid), inositol, biotin and choline. **Because of modern food processing, it is extremely difficult to obtain even the minimum amount of B-Complexes from our food alone.** Current labeling shows the amount of nutrients found in a food before processing, not after. Flour, for example, loses 82% of its B-vitamins in processing, and spaghetti 64%. Even cracked wheat bread has lost 38% of its B-vitamins. A deficiency of just one of the B-vitamins, thiamin causes extreme mood swings due to lack of availability of serotonin, a brain chemical which help regulate emotions. Patients complaining of lethargy, personality changes, and sleep disturbances, lack of appetite, diarrhea, and fevers of unknown origin were studied. These symptoms "would represent a trap for the unwary physician since he would be unable to find any objective physical sign other than variations of normal, which would be easily classed as the effects of a chronic state of anxiety" (American Journal of Clinical Nutrition). When supplemental Thiamin was given, all patients in the study reported a marked symptomatic improvement or a complete loss of all symptoms.

Ingestion of coffee, either regular or decaffeinated, severely depletes Thiamin. Thiamin isn't alone in its ability to affect moods. Niacin depletion causes severe reactions in humans. "If all the niacin were removed from our food, everyone wood be psychotic in one year," (Abram Hoffer, MD and psychiatrist). B-vitamins are also catalysts in the burning of carbohydrates and in glucose tolerance. B-vitamins are water-soluble (Oil-soluble vitamins are A, D, E, and K) so taking them in the morning with breakfast and again with lunch will help insure high energy throughout the day. There are many good quality B-complex supplements for women available in health stores. Be sure to read the labels and understand what you are ingesting. Niacin can cause "flushing" in doses over 30-50mgs, so you may wish to take niacin separately and use a supplement with the "non-flushing" form of niacin, "niacinamide". Niacinamide lacks the beneficial vasodialating effects found in niacin, but "flushing" frightens those who do not understand that flushing is beneficial and is often replaced by niacinamide for that reason.

Chelation and Minerals

Without the proper minerals, vitamins cannot be fully utilized. Minerals are the building blocks for body tissue and other body structures. Minerals enable enzymes and hormones, which regulate the metabolism. Also, minerals maximize the efficiency of healthy essential oils containing the all-important essential fatty acids. Minerals are inorganic and are co-enzymes. Our bodies cannot use raw minerals when taken in their inorganic form because they cannot be digested or used. Plants transform minerals from the soil into an organic form that humans can use by eating vegetables as well as eating animals that have eaten plants and have the minerals present in their meat. The minerals in a supplement should be chelated (bound or "hooked up") to another substance such as an amino acid to promote better bioavailability. Most mineral supplements commonly described as "chelated" have an organic molecule like a citrate or gluconate chemically tied to the mineral, which has a very low bioavailability. Since the intestinal wall readily absorbs proteins, avoid the following so-called chelating agents that are not protein based: citrates, sulfates, gluconates, phosphates, etc.). Chelated minerals are less irritating to the gastrointestinal tract compared to some of the salts of these minerals. We waste money on supplements the body cannot use effectively. For example: By swallowing a 200mg pill of calcium less than 14% is used by the body which translates into 28% bio-availability. Take a 500mg pill of calcium and the body uses almost 70%. How effectively a nutritional supplement is absorbed is far more important than how much is taken. For example: the calcium absorption rate for milk is 30%. For ideal mineral absorption, the ration of minerals to amino acid bonding must be in the ratio between 1-unit of mineral to 3-units of amino acid; the weight of the amino acids in the mineral chelate must be very small (150 Daltons), the total molecular weight must be less than 800 Daltons, and the chelate must not ionize in the digestive system. Digestion quickly separates the commonly used chelating mineral salts or complexes from any mixed-in protein. We want the mineral-protein combination to remain free of positive or negative ions. Otherwise, the mineral will bond with something else and may not be utilized. Note: It is for this reason we suggest that you do not use "Colloidal Minerals!

A mineral plays three roles in the human body:

☆   It supports the energy conversion process

☆   It aids in the growth and maintenance of the body's tissues

☆   They assist in the regulation of all bodily processes.

Contrary to popular belief, chelation does not insure absorption of minerals, as this is best achieved by taking mineral supplements with food containing minerals. The ingestion of fresh food is always the best way to achieve maximum nutrient intake. Individual biochemistry, including enzymatic functions, will generally determine a person's ability to effectively process minerals. However, minerals tied to salts have little bioavailability compared to amino acid chelation. There are 17 minerals, which humans need. The following nine minerals (out of the seventeen) are essential; insofar, as they are not found in our food supply: boron, iron, magnesium, zinc, selenium, copper, manganese, chromium, and potassium. A good mineral supplement should contain the above nine essential minerals, plus calcium, and phosphorus. If the supplement lists all of the minerals in equal doses, opt for another choice, as minerals do not occur in nature in equal amounts. Do not rely on a supplement to supply you with all the minerals you need. Eat fresh vegetables and fruit, beans, fish, turkey and chicken and take a well-formulated vitamin/mineral supplement with fresh food.

Timed-Released

It is better not to use timed-released vitamins. There are exceptions, of course, but they are rare. When it comes to absorption, timed-released nutrients are inferior. Timed-released vitamins are a nice concept, but research shows conclusively that with a timed-released vitamin, the percent of dosage absorbed is low compared to that of a regular non timed-released vitamin. This is especially true of Vitamin-C.

Synergists

Certain vitamins taken without their synergistic sisters are better off not taken at all. No one nutrient occurs in nature all by itself. When Vitamin-C is present in fruit, its sister, the bioflavonoids, always accompanies it. This is extremely important! Minerals occur in nature in certain ratios to each other and they work synergistically, as do the B-vitamins. A good example is cystine. Do not take supplemental cystine without taking at least 3-times as much Vitamin-C as cystine. Taking large amounts of cystine without Vitamin-C can cause cystine stones in the kidneys and urinary bladder. Well made vitamin and mineral supplements are an excellent adjunct to food, but be an informed and aware consumer when choosing your supplements. As you read this book, you will be given valuable information, which is necessary to live a good quality of life. Remember balance and moderation is important too.

Did you know?
Milk is the probable leading cause of Heart Disease?
May lead to an increased risk of breast cancer?
The powerful growth hormones in milk increase the rate of cancer growth.
The body does not adequately absorb calcium in milk.
Milk consumption is the probable cause of osteoporosis.

Chapter 2: Essential Fatty Acids

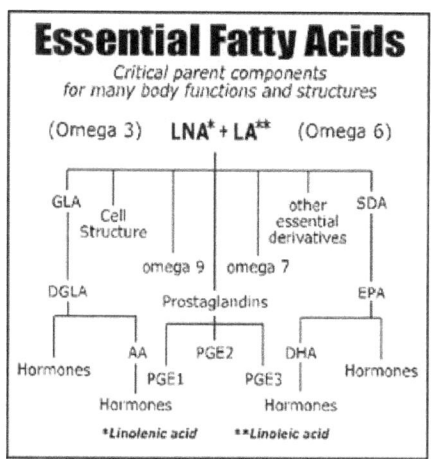

When people say the word "FAT" they immediately think of a food that could add unsightly pounds to their waistline, causing them to gain unnecessary weight. This is just plain wrong! There are "good" fats and "bad" fats and the beneficial ones can actually help decrease the desire to eat the harmful ones. Fats do many things for the body.

Fats, also known as "lipids", are the body's prime source of energy (not carbs).

They balance the body's chemistry and help with the transportation and absorption of fat-soluble vitamins such as vitamins A, D, E, and K. But their most important function is as a source of the vital nutrients known as essential fatty acids (EFAs). Essential Fatty Acids are vital to our body's need for many functions. They are found in seeds of plants and in oils of cold-water fish. EFAs are sometimes referred to as Vitamin F. Since our bodies cannot make EFAs, they must be supplied by our diet. Here is a list of the vital functions EFAs accomplish in our bodies:

☆ Lowers triglyceride levels.

☆ Helps eradicate plaque from arterial walls.

☆ Lowers blood pressure.

☆ Alters the production of leukotrienes, which aggravate inflammation in the body. This is good news to those suffering from arthritis, lupus, psoriasis and other inflammation-related ailments.

☆ Helps to construct body membranes working with cholesterol and protein to repair old cell membranes and construct new ones.

☆ Helps to strengthen cell and capillary structures.

☆ Prolongs blood-clotting time.

☆ Helps in the manufacture of hemoglobin, the compound in the blood that provides oxygen to the cells from the lungs.

☆ Assists in the manufacture of cholesterol and also removes excess cholesterol from the blood. Cholesterol has gotten some undeserved press. Cholesterol is a waxy alcohol and is necessary for many vital bodily functions. Interestingly enough, there is no known cholesterol-sensing mechanism in the body. This tells us that an abundance of cholesterol is not a cause for alarm. It is found in the bile, blood, brain tissue, liver, kidneys, adrenal glands, and the myelin sheath of nerve fibers. It helps absorb and transport EFAs and is necessary for the body to synthesize vitamin D. All hormones are made from cholesterol. The body will actually manufacture cholesterol from dietary by-products of proteins, sugars and fats (by cells, glands, the small intestine and the liver) to insure a continuous supply of this important fat. If your diet contains excessive saturated fats, the body will convert them into cholesterol. People who eat high sugar or fat diets may therefore experience elevated cholesterol levels.

☆ Prevents the growth of bacteria and viruses, which will not thrive in the presence of oxygen, by oxygenating cell membranes. Highly unsaturated fatty acids have the ability to hold oxygen and this results in increasing resistance to disease, increased endurance, better metabolic efficiency and energy conversion, plus the balancing of sleep-wake cycles. And for you workout nuts, EFAs also shorten the recovery times for tired muscles.

☆ Assists in the functions of glands and hormones. (Note: EFAs must be present along with vitamins E and B to produce sex and adrenal hormones.)

☆ Nourishes skin, hair and nails. EFAs help to eliminate eczema, psoriasis, dandruff, and help prevent hair loss.

☆ Increases the rate the body burns fat.

☆ Helps maintain the body's temperature.

☆ Assists in the body's production of electrical currents vital for a regular heartbeat.

☆ Acts as a precursor to the production of hormone-like substances called prostaglandins. Prostaglandins are found in almost all body cells and act as catalysts for many physiological processes. They help prevent abnormal blood clotting and nerve inflammation. Prostaglandins also help promote blood circulation by dilating the blood vessels and improve immune system function. The most beneficial type of prostaglandin is called PGE-1, which balances cholesterol and blood pressure levels, and stimulates the body's production of T-lymphocytes, which strengthen the immune capabilities. Each cell keeps tiny amounts of EFAs and produces prostaglandins from them, as they are needed. The name prostaglandins were coined because these substances were originally found in high amounts in the prostate gland. There are 36 different prostaglandins with a wide range of roles in the body.

"Stress, allergies, disease, and a diet high in fried food, increase the body's need for EFAs"

Let's discuss the types of fats.

Saturated Fats

All fats are composed of carbon, hydrogen, and oxygen molecules. The carbon atoms of fatty acids hold together in a chain-like fashion. These carbon atoms can attach hydrogen to them. When each place that can hold a hydrogen atom is filled and there is no room for even one more atom, they are described as "saturated". The longer the chain, the harder the fat will be and hence, the higher its melting point. These types of "long-chain fatty acids" are found in hard fats such as those in red meat, cheese, sour cream, and palm kernel and coconut oils.

Unsaturated Fats:

These fats are called unsaturated because there are at least two adjacent carbon atoms on a chain, which are not attached to hydrogen atoms. When at least two pairs of carbon atoms are empty, it is known as a monounsaturated fatty acid. When two or more sets are empty, then it is referred to as a polyunsaturated fatty acid. Fatty acids are either essential or nonessential. They are essential if the body cannot synthesize them and the only way they can be obtained is through the diet. As far back as the 1930s, researchers discovered that a lack of EFAs in our diets caused poor reproduction, lowered immunity, rough and dry skin, and slow growth

There are basically three essential fatty acids:

1. Linolenic Acid (Alpha-Lenolenic Omega-3.)

The most common forms of Omega-3 are eicosapentaenioic acid (EPA), docisahexaenoic acid (DHA), and alpha-linolenic acid, which come from plants and help create EPA and DHA. Omega-3 is usually derived from fish oils.

Note: Fish Oils containing Omega-3 found in coldwater fish are salmon, bluefish, herring, tuna, and mackerel.

2. Linoleic Acid (Omega-6)

This is the most vital of the EFAs. The other two, linolenic and arachidonic acids can be converted from linoleic acid. It is plant derived and in its most common form, gamma-linolenic acid (GLA) it is known to provide the following benefits:

☆ Helps facilitate weight loss in overweight persons (but not in people who do not need to lose weight).

☆ Reduces platelet aggregation (abnormal blood clotting).

☆ Helps reduce symptoms of depression and schizophrenia.

☆ Alleviates premenstrual syndrome symptoms.

☆ May help alcoholics overcome their addiction.

Note: Plants that contain Omega-6 are Black Currant Seed Oil, Borage Oils, Flaxseed Oil, and Evening Primrose

3. Arachidonic Acid

Is unique in that it is abundant in brain cells as well as other cells. To the cell membrane, this acid is critical but elsewhere it may not be so beneficial.

EFA Deficiency Symptoms

A lack of Linoleic Acid can cause adverse symptoms including:

- Acne
- Changes in personality or behavior
- Gallbladder dysfunction
- Slow wound healing
- Cardiovascular problems
- Prostate inflammation
- Thirst due to excessive perspiration
- Arthritis
- Miscarriage
- Poor Growth
- Kidney problems
- Muscle Tremors
- Skin disorders
- Sterility in males

A lack of Linolenic Acid can cause adverse symptoms including:

- Poor Growth
- Learning disability
- Tingling in the extremities
- Impaired motor coordination
- Poor Vision

The human body requires forty-five (45) known essential nutrients and it requires linolenic acid (Omega-3) more than any other (at least 6-grams/day). Of the forty-five needed nutrients, 20 are minerals, 15 are vitamins, 8 are amino acids and 2 are fatty acids. Altered fatty acids are called Trans-fatty Acids and are extremely bad for the body. Stay away from deep fried foods. Heated fats, especially of the vegetable kind, may turn into cancer-causing agents by causing free-radical damage to the body. The body CANNOT use trans-fatty acids so they simply collect around fatty tissues and the body's organs. Studies show that EFAs may be helpful for many chronic stubborn conditions. The EFAs' ever growing repertoire of valuable applications includes overcoming diseases such as alcoholism, breast cancer, and cardiovascular disease, strengthening the immune system, helping eliminate yeast infection, reducing symptoms of premenstrual syndrome, minimizing inflammation of rheumatoid arthritis, and assisting in the proper management of weight.

Chapter 3: Did You Know?

DID YOU KNOW?

This section offers some very interesting facts that disprove the prevailing health mindset.

☆ Fat is the body's preferred energy source (not carbs and sugar!). Per unit weight, fats occupy less volume and produce more energy than carbs or protein. One (1) gram of fat produces 2.5 times as much energy as one (1) gram of carbs. We have enough body fat for weeks of survival but only approximately 24-hours of carb reserve.

☆ Insulin stops fat burning even while exercising.

☆ Eating fat does not make you fat. Carbs are stored as fat.

☆ Glucosamine sulfate is not the best thing for joint pain relief because of its effect on inhibiting hepatic glucokinase, the body's glucose sensor.

☆ Attention Deficit Disorder (ADD) and Attention Deficit Hyperactivity Disorder (ADHD) can be reduced by supplementation of Omega 3 and 6 oils. Lack of EPAs contributes to hyperactivity in kids. Boys are much more affected and males need more EFAs than females.

☆ Elevated triglyceride levels (bad) persisted throughout the day induced by high carbs, despite the decrease in fat in the diet. High carb diets are associated with increases in both fasting and postprandial (after eating) triglyceride concentrations.

☆ Substituting carbs for saturated fat leads to higher triglyceride and lower HDL.

☆ The number one health complaint is chronic fatigue.

☆ We consume 160 lbs of sugar per year.

☆ Five (5) grams of carbs equals one (1) teaspoon of sugar. A 12 oz. Can of soda has 35-45 grams of carbs, which equals 7-9 teaspoons of sugar into your bloodstream at one time.

☆ We dump more than 450 teaspoons of sugar into are bloodstreams every week; however our bodies were designed to run on less than 1-teaspoon per week.

☆ 1 pound of body fat equals 3500 stored calories.

- One 8oz. glass of orange juice has enough sugar in it to provide the energy to run one mile.

- The body can manufacture ALL of the carbs it needs from proteins and body fat.

- Eating the right kind of fats reduces body fat

- Carbs are the worst fuel for achieving peak performance

- Carbs stop you from using the fat stored in your own body as the best fuel available.

- In 1900 3% died from heart disease. Today, 46% die from heart disease. The jump in heart disease began in the 1930s; the same decade processed cooking oils began widespread usage. A few years later, margarine replaced butter and processed oils virtually eliminated lard. Today, the average American consumes 10 lbs of chemically processed shortening and 20 lbs of margarine each year.

- Death from heart disease DECREASES 44% with the use of Omega-3 oils.

- If you get food cravings, and frequently run low on energy; if you need 8-hours or more of sleep; if you have cellulite; if you need three meals each day; if you ever feel intensely hungry and/or stressed out, then you fail the healthy eating test.

- The cause of plaque build-up in the arteries are tiny cuts or wounds to the arterial wall caused by insulin whereas the body, needing to repair these cuts, places cholesterol as a "scab" eventually leading to a build-up or blockage called plaque.

- Presumably, the cholesterol in the LDL, coming from the liver to the tissues, is more likely to be deposited at the sites of the arterial wall lesions and cholesterol in the HDL, traveling to the liver, is less likely to contribute to the lesion. Hence LDL cholesterol has the label "bad" and HDL cholesterol has the label "good".

- The only reason we are eating so many calories is because food processing removes or destroys essential nutrients, triggering the body to signal hunger in hope of getting what it needs.

- The human gut is proportionately many times longer than that of a strict carnivore. Humans have a weaker stomach acid concentration (10-times weaker than a carnivore). Carnivores need a shorter, more powerful gut to quickly digest raw meat, bone and feathers. Humans are omnivores.

- Fresh fish has NO smell and tastes buttery. A fishy smell is a sign that the EFAs are going bad.

- This is something to take into consideration: Virtually all research is conducted on test subjects that are EFA-deficient.

- The female breast contains a very high proportion of fat cells. Our bodies tend to concentrate and store toxins in fat tissues; hence, we should expect toxins from the air, water and food to build up in a woman's breast tissue, which may cause the increase in breast cancer.

☆ Genetic problems are not the cause of obesity. A gene cannot act by itself; it must combine with other genes to produce a noticeable trait and even then, a gene only presents tendency. They do not dictate actions. Since there is no known genetic cause for obesity, there is no need for medical intervention. Since the problem has a nutritional root, it must be solved by a nutrition-related solution. This is why drug companies need to step back from offering a medical-related solution. Being drugged for a lifetime is not the solution.

☆ The body has to quickly convert carbs to fat because toxic by-products are formed during the cell's use and breakdown of glucose. If these by-products cannot be used by the body fast enough, they are converted directly to fat and cholesterol to protect us from self-poisoning.

☆ This is really going to shock you. Studies show that vigorous exercise offers virtually no additional mortality protection over moderate exercise. When your body has the optimal amount of EFAs, your endurance increases and exercise becomes easier.

☆ A person burns 10-times as much glucose doing anaerobic exercise compared to the same amount of aerobic exercise.

☆ It would take 10-hours of walking or 5-hours of aerobics to burn 1-pound of body fat.

☆ A person eating 20% carbs/ 80% protein and natural fats after just 10-minutes of aerobics is burning 50% of energy from body fat. After 1-hour it is 65%!

☆ A typical government recommended diet of 2000 calories/day contains as much as 1200 calories from carbs, which is equivalent to 60-teaspoons of sugar.

☆ If you are thin and consume large quantities of food without weight gain, beware; this is often the main symptom of the onset of diabetes because the person is not metabolizing much of the food. A glycohemoglobin test will detect diabetes.

☆ Salt is required for cellular sugar transfer.

☆ Our brain feeds on glucose and uses two-thirds of the circulating glucose in the bloodstream.

☆ A typical 180 lb male has 15% body fat or 27 pounds. Twenty-percent (5-7 Pounds) is used structurally throughout the body, so approximately 20 pounds of fat is excess body fat called adipose tissue. A typical 130-pound female has 22% body fat or 29 pounds.

☆ There is a big difference between thriving and surviving

☆ Only 1% of your pancreas can be used to make insulin. The other 99% is involved in other various digestive processes. The pancreas is not a muscle like the heart, which works continuously. It is designed to secrete insulin once or twice a day in response to carbohydrates with several hours between secretions. Is it any wonder with the high carb diets that we have virtually worn our pancreas out?

☆ By taking EFAs 20-30-minutes before meals means you'll desire less food.

☆ Here's a real shocker: More than two-thirds of all the deaths reported in the United States involves nutrition.

- When you eat natural fat, it goes directly into your lymphatic system-NOT into the bloodstream. A protein must be placed around the fat before it enters the bloodstream. There is no loose fat running around in your bloodstream.

- An average 130-pound female requires a full pound of protein per day for normal body processes. This could be in the form of a high quality whey protein powder but preferably food.

- More than 50% of your body weight is protein. Amino acids are made from protein.

- There are 20 amino acids. The human body can produce 11 of these. That leaves 9, which are called essential amino acids: Histidine, Lysine, Threonine, Isoleucine, methionine, Tryptophan, Leucine, Phenylalanine, and Valine.

- Triglycerides are fat made from carbohydrates.

- Salt is not bad for you! If you eat too much salt, the body's equilibrium systems go into action and counteract it, i.e. "The Atrial Naturietic Factor" (ANF), which triggers kidneys to dump sodium. Human cells contain almost 1% salt-based nutrients. Stomach acid requires chloride from salt.

- For deep-frying use peanut oil or coconut oil. For all other cooking use olive oil. Tropical oils do not raise cholesterol levels.

- Brown age spots or "liver" spots are indicative of degeneration in the body. EFAs cause them to become lighter or disappear.

- Women taking oral contraceptives and exercising have a significantly higher risk of developing a prethrombic (blood clot) condition.

- Here is another shocker: Osteoporosis is not caused by a lack of calcium in the bloodstream. The following are the causes: Lack of physical stress on the bone from inactivity, shortage of protein, lack of vitamin C, postmenopausal lack of estrogen, decrease in growth hormone (HGH) and other hormones inhibiting bone matrix, and Cushings disease (adrenal tumor)

- Never use hormone supplements unless prescribed. A tiny bit of hormone causes drastic changes in the body. All hormone production typically decreases with age. Many hormones (and all postaglandins) are made from EFAs.

- DHEA is converted in the body into androgens and other steroid hormones.

- The definition for appetite is the desire for food; hunger is the need for food.

- The myth of increasing the metabolism to burn more fat wrongly implies that the body is a heat engine when the truth is that it is a chemical engine.

- RDA for fat is 65 grams/day based on a 2000 cal/day diet.

Chapter 4: Cellulite

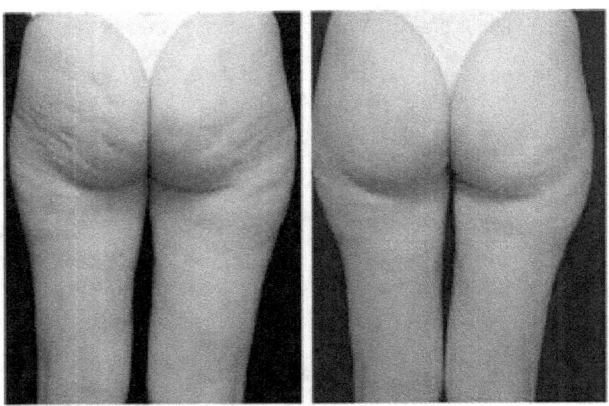

CELLULITE is the scourge of women's thighs and the bane of the female swimsuit industry that causes clothing executives to place their head in their hands and speak in tongues. Without a doubt the most often asked question of the beauty industry today is, **"How do I get rid of cellulite?"** To begin to answer the question, let's define what cellulite is. Cellulite is an accumulation of fat globules trapped between the muscle and the skin. If allowed to go unchecked, the fat globules may increase in size and compaction and the result: a quasi-armor plating of fat that robs women of their self-esteem and causes untold misery to millions of American women. Now that you know what cellulite is, let's define what it IS NOT:

☆   Cellulite IS NOT related to excess body fat.

☆   Cellulite IS NOT related to the ingestion of fat in our diets. ELIMINATING DIETARY FAT DOES NOTHING TO CONTROL CELLULITE. Thin women have it as well as obese women.

☆   Cellulite IS NOT treated by strenuous aerobic exercise. Marathon runners and female bodybuilders have cellulite.

☆   Cellulite IS NOT caused by fluid trapped in the tissues.

☆   Cellulite IS NOT eliminated by vigorous massage.

☆   Cellulite is NOT eliminated by eating high fiber diets and/or diuretic foods (cucumbers, celery, and grapefruit).

Although cellulite most often appears on a woman's upper rear thighs, it can appear elsewhere. It is also now known that cellulite does have a hereditary nature. Cellulite can and does appear on men but it appears less because men have thicker skin. In fact, women have 20%

thinner skin than men but have a whopping 50% more body fat. We also know that a high carbohydrate diet does increase cellulite build-up by increasing the Advanced Glycosycation end-products (AGEs) in the body. These AGEs cross link with proteins and act like little magnets. It is this opposite polarity magnetic effect that causes the hill-and-valley ripple look of cellulite. AGES are known to build-up and cause problems with arteries and DNA. WHAT IS THE CAUSE OF CELLULITE? Answer: Cellulite's main cause is the lack of essential fatty acids in your diet.

Let's discuss cellulite's annoying hill-and-valley structure. Most of our diets consist of highly processed oils and fats. From these processed oils and fats come Transfatty Acids (TFAs). These TFAs have replaced the necessary and needed essential fatty acids (EFAs) which are body thrives on but of which we obtain very little of in our diets because of the highly processed foods that we consume. Furthermore, these TFAs are not as flexible within the cell wall as the EFAs that they have replaced. Their rigidity interferes with the natural cell flexibility. The lack of cell flexibility magnifies the hill-and-valley effect. Cellulite is an EFA deficiency indicator. By understanding the human body, one will see that many problems relate to nutrition. Women especially have different dietary needs than a man. Without a proper diet, women can develop very serious problems. There are some skeletal differences worth mentioning here. A woman's spine is shorter than a man's spine by about an inch. This is because of childbearing. Also, a woman's pelvis is wider than a man's pelvis and is the reason for the "wiggle" in a woman's walk. It is these two skeletal differences that cause a woman to accumulate fat on her thighs, especially her rear thighs since it is the least problematic area for the body to deposit fat. A bipedal (two legged) animal has the ability to stand upright by a unique sense of balance found in our inner ear. If the skeleton is misaligned, due to trauma or childbirth, the body will adjust for balance by placing fat in problem areas. In a woman, the adjustment usually occurs in the thighs. Men, being much larger and taller than a woman and consequently having a higher center of gravity, have the adjustment usually centered in the gut area. Treatment of unsightly cellulite is relatively easy by using the "Fit-4-Life" Complete Health System Protocol described in Chapter 8.

Chapter 5: The Glycemic Index and HGH

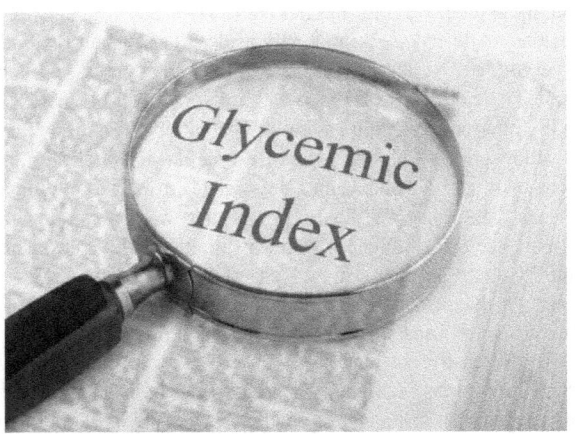

I want to steer you into a new nutritional thought pattern, one that is "contrary" to the accepted "parroted" line that high carbohydrate/low fat and protein diets are what is best for optimum health. If you believe this then you really need to read this report.

The "Fit-4-Life" Complete Health System utilizes the principle that optimum health is achieved when the mind-body-soul are at their peak of efficiency. We achieve the body side of the equation by replacing the essential fatty acids that the high carbohydrate/low fat diets have removed. The American people are addicted to carbohydrates due to the highly processed nature of our food supply.

In addition, the "Fit-4-Life" Complete Health System utilizes a mineral supplement that replaces the nine essential minerals that are not found in our food supply. Furthermore, the program calls for a detoxifying tea that removes the accumulation of toxins from the body. As the body releases its excess fat stores, the toxins, which are stored in the adipose (fat) tissues, are released.

Last, our program utilizes a Human Growth Hormone (HGH) precursor formulation and it is this we will now address.

Human Biochemistry, Human Growth Hormone and Positive Nitrogen Balance

Positive nitrogen balance is achieved by having more amino acids going into the body than going out. Excess amino acids are stored as fat unless there is HGH present. The equation looks like this:

Excess amino acids + HGH =Muscle

Excess amino acids - HGH = Stored Fat

To increase the release of HGH by the pituitary gland naturally there must be an increase in physical exercise, an increase in sleep plus the biochemical response to a HGH precursor formulation, which is widely available on the health market today. Release of HGH plus your low carb diet equals: increased lean muscle mass, increased strength, reduced body fat, steady anabolic rate and increased endurance. HGH determines whether dietary protein is converted to fat or muscle. If you want to add lean muscle mass, you will have to exercise, stimulate HGH with an HGH precursor formulation, decrease total carbohydrate consumption to low or moderate glycemic carbs and increase the intake of properly balanced proteins and minerals and fat. Yes I said FAT! Contrary to popular belief, **the body's preferred energy source is not carbohydrates. It is FAT!**

What is the difference between high and low glycemic carbs? Diet and exercise should be directed at increasing natural HGH. HGH is inhibited by insulin and is contraindicated to excess insulin.

Ratios of HGH to insulin determine ratios of lean body mass to body fat.

High HGH ratios to insulin result in lean muscularity, while low ratios of HGH to insulin result in excess body fat. Foods high in the glycemic index raise blood sugar, which triggers insulin to be released by the pancreas, which in turn causes calories for carbs to be stored as body fat.

So **high glycemic carbs inhibit HGH and exacerbate the storage of fat.**

High glycemic carbs can also cause reactive hypoglycemia evidenced by weakness and fatigue. The glycemic index rates foods according to their ability to raise blood sugar levels. **Low glycemic carbs do not interrupt HGH release or add fat calories.**

Why haven't we heard about the glycemic index before?

The American Diabetic Association and doctors working in the field of diabetes have been using the glycemic index for almost 20-years. The index has been updated in 1986, 1990 and 1991.

How does the glycemic index relate to my muscle to fat ratio?

When you ingest carbohydrates, the pancreas secretes insulin. Conversely, when you ingest protein, the pancreas releases glucagon. It is insulin's job to remove sugar form the blood by pushing it into cells. Excess sugar overwhelms the pancreas and the sugar is simply "swept under the rug" by putting into fat cells. In attempting to promote muscle size and strength gains, too many high glycemic carbs and sugars are generally consumed. When too much insulin is released due to eating too many high glycemic carbs, the body becomes overly efficient in storing calories. When this process occurs over and over, the body does not easily relinquish its fat stores. A good HGH precursor formulation should contain: L-Arginine, 100% free-form, 6 grams per serving, 30 servings to a bottle, 667 mgs of choline, branched chain aminos, fructose, boron, pantothenic acid (B-5), calcium pantothenate, chromium polynicotinate. Note: cannot contain L-Lysine or any other protein.

Foods Low in the Glycemic Index

 Apples

☆ Applesauce

☆ Asparagus

☆ Baked Beans

☆ Barbecue Ribs

☆ Beef

☆ Black-Eyed Peas

☆ Blueberries

☆ Broccoli

☆ Buttermilk

☆ Cabbage

☆ Cantaloupe

☆ Cauliflower

☆ Celery

☆ Cherries

☆ Chicken

☆ Chickpeas

☆ Cucumber

☆ Dried Peas

☆ Egg Roll

☆ Fried Chicken

☆ Fried Fish

☆ Garlic

☆ Grapefruit

☆ Grapes

☆ Green Beans

☆ Green Chilies

☆ Green Peppers

☆ Honey Dew Melon

- ☆ Ice Cream
- ☆ Kidney Beans
- ☆ Leeks
- ☆ Lemon
- ☆ Lentils
- ☆ Lettuce
- ☆ Lima Beans
- ☆ Lime
- ☆ Milk
- ☆ Mushrooms
- ☆ Nuts
- ☆ Oatmeal
- ☆ Oranges
- ☆ Peaches
- ☆ Peanuts
- ☆ Pears
- ☆ Pepper Steak
- ☆ Plums
- ☆ Pork Rinds
- ☆ Radishes
- ☆ Raspberries
- ☆ Red Bell Peppers
- ☆ Sauerkraut
- ☆ Scallions
- ☆ Seeds
- ☆ Snow Peas
- ☆ Soy Beans
- ☆ Spinach

Sponge Cake

 Squash

 Steamed Fish

 Strawberries

 Sweet Potato

 Tangerine

 Tomato

 Yogurt (Frozen)

 Zucchini

Foods Neutral in the Glycemic Index

 Bacon

 Butter

 Cheese

 Coffee

 Egg Whites

 Ground Beef

 Hot Dogs

 Jell-O

 Lamb

 Olive Oil

 Parmesan

 Peanut Butter

 Pork Chops

 Sausage

 Seafood (Not Fried)

 Steak

 Tuna

- ☆ Turkey
- ☆ Venison
- ☆ Vinegar
- ☆ Whole Eggs

Foods Moderate in the Glycemic Index

- ☆ Artichokes
- ☆ Avocado
- ☆ Beets
- ☆ Chocolate Milk
- ☆ Colas
- ☆ Cookies
- ☆ Mayonnaise
- ☆ Orange Juice
- ☆ Pasta
- ☆ Pastries
- ☆ Pineapple
- ☆ Pita Bread
- ☆ Pizza
- ☆ Raisins
- ☆ Spaghetti
- ☆ Sugar
- ☆ Watermelon
- ☆ Wheat Tortillas

Foods High in the Glycemic Index

- ☆ Banana
- ☆ Brown Rice

- ☆ Candy
- ☆ Carrots
- ☆ Cereal
- ☆ Corn
- ☆ Corn Chips
- ☆ Glucose
- ☆ Honey
- ☆ Oat Bran
- ☆ Pancakes And Syrup
- ☆ Parsnips
- ☆ Potato
- ☆ Potato Chips
- ☆ Puffed Rice
- ☆ Rice Cakes
- ☆ Rolled Oats
- ☆ Wheat Bread
- ☆ White Bread
- ☆ White Rice

Chapter 6: Candida Albicans

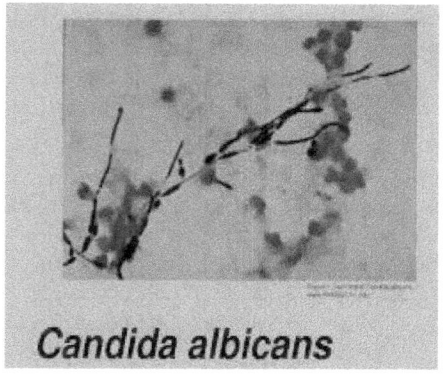

Candida albicans

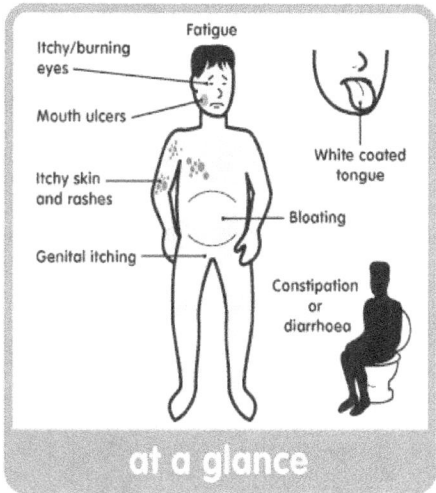

at a glance

Candida overgrowth

(For women and men)

The world is a very tough place. Each and every one of us lives in a sea of bacteria. Infectious agents, known as microbes, swim daily throughout our bodies. Microbes can reside in our throat, mouth, gums, nose, gastrointestinal tract, etc. These microorganisms (i.e., bacteria, viruses, and fungi) are as much a part of every human being as foods and chemicals that we ingest daily. Figuratively speaking, they are constantly trying to "eat us alive". Sometimes they succeed! Even if we die of causes other than infection, they eventually eat our physical remains. Only healthy cells, tissues and organs within our bodies can effectively defend against infectious microorganisms and these make up what is called our immune system.

Microbes, whether they are bacteria, viruses or fungi, do not usually cause illness until an individual's host resistance declines. "Host resistance" is a technical term used by physicians to describe the complicated mechanisms by which our bodies fight off infections. One of the most important defense mechanisms is the destruction of invading microorganisms by blood leukocytes (white blood cells). These special cells actually ingest microbes and render them harmless. But before leukocytes can be manufactured in the body, there must be an optimum supply of amino acids, vitamins A, C, B1, B2, B6, B12 biotin, niacinamide, pantothenic acid and others as well as a complete balance of all minerals and trace elements. If even a single amino acid is deficient or missing, leukocyte production is diminished or may even cease. When this occurs, host resistance within the body is weakened and a greater susceptibility to infection of all kinds ensues.

Another host resistance defense mechanism is the antibody system. When our bodies are receiving optimal nutritional support, specialized protein substances known as antibodies are produced. These substances are constructed from chains of amino acids (proteins). Antibodies also attack invading microorganisms and render them susceptible to destruction by the leukocytes. An individual infectious microbe always provokes antibodies that are specifically targeted against that particular type of microbe and no other. Once the body has synthesized specific antibodies, the lymph cells can reproduce them any time they are needed, provided there are optimum levels of amino acids, vitamins, minerals, trace elements and enzymes from which they can be constructed. Accordingly, if your antibodies for measles, for example, have been synthesized, you will more than likely remain free of measles upon re-exposure to the measles virus. In such a case, your host resistance (i.e., a healthy immune system or adequate production of antibodies, leukocytes and phagocytes), maintained via optimum nutritional support, is functioning properly.

It is essential to understand, therefore, that in the real world, infectious illness occurs not because some "germ" arbitrarily decides to attack our bodies. Rather, illness occurs because our nutritionally deficient, debilitated bodies permit these microbes to set up residence. In short, an opportunist microbe is an infectious agent that produces disease only when the circumstances are favorable.

Nutrient deficits can severely impair the integrity of a healthy immune system. Other factors, however, are also critically involved in resistance to infection. The ingestion of large amounts of sugar, for example, paralyzes the phagocytic capacity of our white blood cells. Likewise, when you fail to obtain your needed quota of sleep, resistance to infectious invasion decreases. Similarly, a personal loss, chronic constipation or diarrhea, irritative chemical exposures to respiratory epithelium, anxiety, too much physical stress, chronic food-chemical allergies and other factors can all influence your resistance to infections. Yet underlying all of these possible causes of poor health are specific nutrient deficiencies, which must be individually tested and diagnosed, and then treated according to empirical laboratory findings.

Traditional medical treatment for bacterial infections flare-up is the administration of antibiotics. Usually little or no advice is given to the patient concerning nutritional support for weakened resistance. And although traditional treatment generally involves drugs that allay symptomatic disorders, the use of drugs does not cure the underlying nutritional-metabolic deficiencies, which are usually the fundamental cause of the illness in the first place. To be sure, this is not to argue against the use of antibiotics. At times, they are very helpful and necessary. However, if the nutritional root causes of infectious disease are not treated, illness after illness may continue to occur, and often become worse, as time goes on. To make matters more disquieting, typical antibiotic medical treatment aimed at the symptomatic relief of infectious flare-up does in fact sometimes produce serious side effects in the form of fungal disorders. The microorganism Candida Albicans is one prevalent example of an infectious overgrowth resulting from the repetitive use, or misuse, of antibiotics.

In its current incarnation, Candida seems to strike women more often than men. Because of the warm, moist condition of the vagina, that is the area most commonly affected. As is the case with all other forms of infection, a compromised host resistance is the primary cause of Candida Albicans. The problem occurs when there is an abnormal fungus, yeast, growth that is normally controlled by friendly bacteria in the intestines. When factors such as antibiotics, steroids (like cortisone), birth control pills and refined sugar are used in excess, friendly bacteria and/or specific nutrients in the blood are destroyed. Host resistance is then lowered and the yeast fungi begin to invade and colonize the body's cells, tissues and finally the organs. A strong, healthy immune systems will, of course, contain Candida's growth. When colonized, these yeast fungi release toxic chemicals into the blood and cause such varying symptoms as yeast vaginitis, rectal itching, chronic diarrhea or constipation, menstrual cramps and irregularities, bladder infections, lethargy, headaches, acne, severe depression, anxiety, nervousness, mental confusion and others. Toxic chemicals produced by the Candida fungi attack the immune system, permitting the fungi to continue their tissue invasion and to cause more serious symptomatic disorders.

Diagnosis

In order to confirm the presence of candidiasis, one must have a high index of suspicion of the condition. Recognition of the risk factors that predispose one to Candida overgrowth is helpful. These are:

☆ Pregnancy or multiple pregnancies.

☆ History of taking birth control pills.

☆ Diabetes mellitus.

☆ History of taking cortisone (corticosteroids).

☆ History of taking antibiotics, especially those of the tetracycline type.

☆ Chemotherapy, irradiation, prolonged illness, debilitation, malnutrition, indwelling catheters, hyperalimentation.

☆ A diet high in sweets, fruits, and juices.

☆ The presence of multiple food allergies and chemical sensitivities.

Candidiasis is the medical term used to describe the yeast fungus overgrowth. It is by no means a new medical problem. In fact, it has been around for centuries. However, candidiasis has become a chronic modern medical dilemma that seems to be increasing rapidly. The reasons for this are the declining vitality of many persons because of several generations of sub optimal diets and the associated factors of drug and chemical exposures.

Treatment

Treatment of candidiasis can involve four major steps: First, the yeast fungi must be killed using a drug called Nystatin. Second, all immuno-suppressive drugs and antibiotics must be used only when necessary. Third, the diet can be altered to deprive the yeast of food upon which it flourishes. Fourth, and most important of all, the body's weakened nutritionally based immune system must be strengthened and thus restored to its proper function. Other forms of treatment are available for those who either cannot tolerate Nystatin or wish not to take the drug. Ketoconazole is a broad-spectrum antifungal drug. Natural treatments include:

☆ Douche twice a day with a mixture of one-pint water to which is added 4 aqueous chlorophyll capsules and 1 tablespoon of vinegar.

☆ At bedtime, insert 2-Zymex wafers in the vagina and wear a pad to keep them in place. Zymex wafers contain a strain of yeast known as lactic acid yeast that inhibits Candida.

☆ Lactobacillus acidophilus organisms can also be inserted in the vagina to counter Candida. Care must be taken that only potent live cultures of Lactobacilli are used,

☆ Intervaginal use of herbs can also effectively combat vaginal Candida infection. One such herbal powder consists of a mixture of squaw vine, chickweed, slippery elm, comfrey, yellow dock, golden seal, mullein and marshmallow. These treatments must, of course, be undertaken only with the permission and supervision of a physician.

☆ Garlic also kills Candida. Garlic can be taken fresh or in the odorless form orally. Olive oil and the B vitamin biotin also suppress Candida.

☆ Low carbohydrate (20%)/high protein (50%)/high fat (30%) diet.

☆ Prohibition of all foods containing yeast such as cheeses, bread, sour cream, buttermilk, beer, wine, cider, mushrooms, soy sauce, tofu, vinegar, dried fruits, melons, and frozen or canned juices.

☆ Inclusion of flaxseed oil (four 1000 mg gel caps) taken in the morning and the evening.

☆ A mineral supplement chelated to amino acids only.

Chapter 7: New Cancer Gene Research

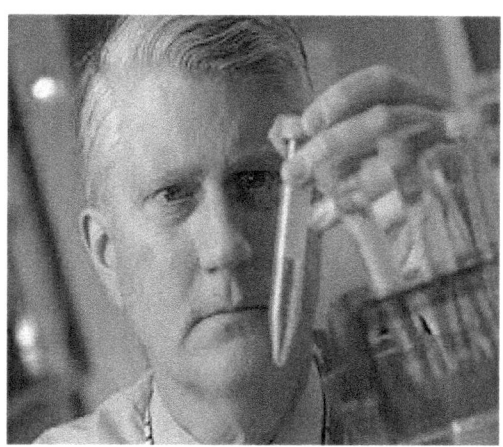

Cancer-the most dreaded word in the English language!

Americans have watched cancer statistics steadily rise to frightening proportions. We all know someone who has fought cancer and lost the battle: Healthy people, young people, and athletes.

No one is exempt from the rising cancer rate.

What is the common denominator linking those destined to develop malignant cells?

Scientific speculation includes diet, exercise, environment, pollution, stress, genetics, and the combination of all of these factors.

☆ Are the excesses of a modern society relative to the growing cancer rate?

☆ What is causing the national cancer rate to accelerate from one-in-five, to one-in-four, to one-in-three, despite millions of dollars of research?

☆ Cancer treatment protocols are becoming more effective, but what about identifying specific causal relationships?

☆ If scientists cannot identify specific causes, how can we hope to effect preventative measures?

☆ If the cancer rate continues to rise unchecked, are we, as a race, destined to develop cells, which mutate in response to our changing society and environment? It is an issue that must be dealt with on a medical, psychological, and financial level.

☆ Smoking has been positively linked to lung cancer, but what explains case histories of eighty-year-old men with a thirty-year history of smoking two packs a day of unfiltered cigarettes and no incidence of lung disease? Is it possible that we inherit the ability to ward off cancer?

☆ Do our genes protect us from malignancies that would develop in someone who did not possess the protective genes?

Our DNA is made up of literally billions of "letters".

Clues that signal genetic mistakes hide within this mega mass of letters.

Gene hunters are scientists trained to track down these well-hidden clues.

They look for markers in chromosomes, which indicate, inherited disease.

Detecting the altered genetic sequence would allow for early removal of malignant cells, cells that are so small they can be removed by simple needle biopsy.

If we can control inherited mutated genes, can we stop all forms of cancer from growing?

No, because 90% of cancers are caused by gene mutation related to our environment.

The leading causes may include smoking, herbicides and pesticides sprayed on the food supply, chemicals in the air and water, and radiation.

The other 10% of cancers are genetically inherited. Research scientists have proven that the on/off switch for cancer cells is within us at all times and is found in the genes that program our cells.

Until methodologies are perfected which control the growth of cancer cells from gene defects related or environmental causes, the best treatment is prevention.

Given the vast amount of scientific data linking free radicals and cancer, it would be wise to adopt a sound preventative program that includes:

☆ A low carbohydrate (30%) / high protein diet.

☆ Daily exercise to stimulate immune function.

☆ Keep abdominal body fat levels low. Hormones in the fat cells contribute to cancer.

☆ Eat a fair amount of dietary fiber.

☆ Avoid direct sunlight and use sunscreen.

☆ Take free radical scavengers daily.

☆ Be aware of any changes in your body.

☆ Become familiar with your gene pool.

☆ Avoid stressful lifestyles

☆   Do not smoke.

You should be aware of some interesting research involving skin cancer in mice.

A gene-called NM-23-when it is found to be normal within the cell apparently prevents the spread of cancer. In cancers that metastasized, the NM-23 gene was defective.

It was obvious that the NM-23 gene was involved in preventing the metastatic process, but exactly how it worked was a mystery.

The hypothesis is that the gene is able to control the spread of cancer cells by acting like a sort of biological glue.

When the activity of the NM-23 gene is turned off, tumor cells spread very quickly.

When the gene is functional, the cancer cells stay glued together.

This startling data represents a significant genetic breakthrough.

Chapter 8: "Fit-4-Life" Complete Health System Protocol

Please Note: The information provided below is for educational purposes only and is not recommended as a means of diagnosing or treating a physical or mental illness or condition. All matters concerning physical or mental health should be supervised by a health practitioner. Although this regimen utilizes only natural supplements, we recommend you notify your health practitioner prior to beginning any new diet regimen.

Exclusively for: _____ Start Date: _____/_____/_____

Beginning Weight: _____lbs. Target Weight: _____lbs. Age: _____

This Lifestyles Regimen Program involves the following supplements:

Natural Organic Oils (1,000 mgs gel caps recommended) made from a variety of natural oils such as flaxseed, sesame, sunflower, etc. containing:

☆ Alpha-Linolenic Acid/Omega-3

☆ Linoleic Acid/Omega-6

☆ Oleic Acid/Omega-9

Any health food store carries flaxseed oil gel caps. A fair price for 200-count is approximately $15-$16.00. Make sure, by reading the label on the bottle that it is 1,000 mgs, that it contains the three above Omega 3, 6, 9 ingredients. Also, keep the open bottle refrigerated. **Directions: take 3-capsules in the morning 30-minutes before eating and 3-capsules in the evening 30-minutes before eating.**

Comprehensive Mineral Supplement (amino acid chelated) containing the following nine essential minerals: boron, iron, magnesium, zinc, selenium, copper, manganese, chromium, potassium, as well as containing the following key ingredients: molybdenum, l-glutamic acid,

MSM (methylsulfonylmethane), horsetail extract, sulfer, vanadium, phosphorus, and calcium. Make sure the mineral supplement is amino acid chelated!!! If it is not, you are wasting your money. Furthermore, make sure it contains the above nine essential minerals. The word "essential" means that they are not obtained in your diet and are needed as a supplement. **Directions: Take two (2) tablets daily.**

Detoxification Tea containing the following certified organic ingredients: burdock root, sheep sorrel herb, slippery elm bark, watercress herb, Turkish rhubarb root, blessed thistle herb, and red clover blossom. I recommend Flor*Essence Herbal Life-Giving Tea, 2.2 oz (Makes 3 quarts of tea) for $21.99. This is an Esiac formulation and is of superior quality. Also, this is the dry formula that you make yourself and is a very good value. **Directions: Follow manufacturer's instructions to make tea as well as dosage amount.**

HGH Supplement: an amino acid based precursor that causes the pituitary gland to secrete more human growth hormone.

☆ Do not take any additional supplements without prior notification of Lifestyle Visions.

☆ Limit ingestion of carbohydrates to 20% of a total dietary intake of 2,000 calories/day. 1 gram of carbs =1tsp. of sugar = 5 calories.

☆ Light exercise (anaerobic is preferred) is recommended.

Chapter 9: Somatotype Body Types / Metabolisms

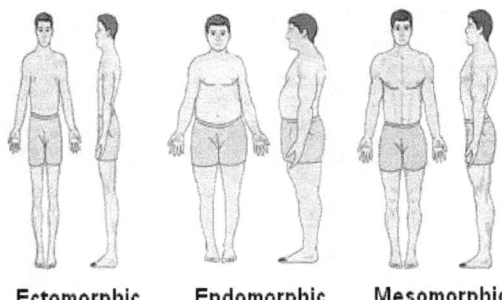

Ectomorphic   Endomorphic   Mesomorphic

Description and Questionnaire

Human Body Types

Endomorph

The Endomorph body type can build muscle successfully but will have to do so by using atypical methods. For example, the usual methods of bodybuilding do not work well for the Endomorph, due to his genetic propensity to store fat. "Work smarter, not harder" should be the motto of the Endomorph for he can get 100% faster and better results by understanding his own biochemistry. Typical dieting and training will bring frustration to the Endomorph. He sees himself going by-the-book in diet and training, but just not getting the right results. The Endomorph is more psychologically tied to food, and to tell an Endomorph not to eat when he is hungry defies what his brain is telling him to do. The Endomorph will need to eat more low glycemic foods than any other body type as he will store fat very easily and will find it difficult to lose weight without starving. Dropping calories will not work for the Endomorph, as the calories he craves, modifies his temperament. Instead of deprivation, the Endomorph should eat when he is hungry - just eat the right foods. No high or moderately high glycemic foods; i.e., sucrose, bananas, or raisins as they exacerbate the Endomorph's fat storing tendencies. Aerobic exercise will be the key factor for the Endomorph bodybuilder. He will have to run, bike; take aerobics, etc. to hold a very low body fat level. Swimming should be avoided by the Endomorph, as it will add body fat (unless the Endomorph is a very heavy swimmer). The Endomorph endurance athlete won't have a problem with extra body fat until he stops training. The Endomorph bodybuilder, or strength athlete, will achieve success by following a regimen of high-sets and high-reps combined with 30-minutes of aerobic exercise every day and a very low glycemic diet of no less than 1,800 calories per day.

Mesomorph

The Mesomorph is the most muscular of all the Somatotypes. He naturally has some muscle whether he exercises or not. The typical Mesomorph has a thick muscle structure, a large chest, thick arms and legs, and is extremely strong. The Mesomorph can build muscle easily and with the right diet can become massive as well as ripped. The key for the Mesomorph body type in bodybuilding is diet. He possesses all the physical basics, so it is just a matter of chiseling down the sculpture to the proper dimensions. The Mesomorph can easily hold too much water, and needs to move that water into the muscle and out of the subcutaneous fat so he looks large and defined. He can only accomplish this through diet and not by any exercise or weightlifting program alone. Obviously an excellent weight-training program is essential, but to the Mesomorph, diet is number one! He has already been blessed genetically, which makes his muscles respond quickly to training. The Mesomorph must eat more protein than the other two body types. His ancestors, Australopithecus Africanus, were hunters and gatherers, and as such, consumed as much live protein as they could catch. Trying to change thousands of years of genetic programming is a waste of time.

The bodybuilding Mesomorph needs to maintain his constant weight (within 10 lbs.) year round. He needs to eat 30 to 50 grams of high quality, lean protein as food and/or acceptable weight gain powders, 5-6 times a day. Ingesting more than around 50 grams of protein at one time is counter-productive and will not result in more lean muscle mass. A Mesomorph should not attempt to hold the same body fat level as an ectomorph. The latest data reflects that in many Mesomorphs, ingesting less than 30% fat in their diet results in the Mesomorph muscle "flattening out". This means manipulating the type of fats in the Mesomorph diet is much more important than simply reducing the total fat intake to the typically recommended 15% to 20%. The high oleic monounsaturated fats should replace the polyunsaturated and saturated fats. The Mesomorph bodybuilder should consume 1 gram of lean protein for every pound of lean muscle mass (not total weight). This should be eaten with cruciferous vegetables (for proper metabolism of protein) and low to moderate glycemic carbs for a total daily intake of not less than 2200 balanced calories.

Ectomorph

The Ectomorph will need to take in more calories than most body types, as their metabolism is so efficient it burns up food easily and effectively. They usually have to eat consistently to gain weight, and may be underweight. Properly formulated weight gain powders are usually required to add muscle mass to the Ectomorph. What the ectomorph does not need is sucrose or glucose in foods, supplements or weight gainers as those types of sugars tend to make his abdominal region round and soft. Ectomorphs are usually extremely flexible. They also make excellent long distance runners. In training, an Ectomorph will need to work harder to build maximum muscle, and will need a lot of sleep (8-10 hours per night). If they are not gaining muscle, then caloric and total nutrient intake will need to increase and they will need to eat more frequently. Unlike the other body types, the Ectomorph can usually eat as much food as he desires and not gain weight. That same metabolic blessing becomes a problem when attempting to add muscle mass. An Ectomorph can usually eat more high glycemic foods than the other two body types and not gain body fat. If an Ectomorph is gaining too much body fat as they work to gain muscle, they can eat foods lower in the glycemic index. For an Ectomorph, they key to gaining muscle mass is to steadily increase their total daily intake of calories until muscle mass is evidenced. Ectomorphs have been known to consume from 8,000 to 10,000 calories per day before gaining substantial muscle mass. In bodybuilding Ectomorphs, very intense weight training balanced with long rest periods is essential. Aerobic exercise should be kept to a minimum, as an Ectomorph who gets a lot of aerobic exercise can easily develop a body profile of 98% lean mass with 2% body fat. The Ectomorph will feel lethargic if he does not get exercise of some type at least three times per week. For cardiovascular fitness, using the Stairmaster or swimming for 1/2 hour, three times per week, would suit the Ectomorph's system.

Human Maximum Performance Somatotypes Questionnaire

Somatotypes

The three different body types: Mesomorph, Endomorph, and Ectomorph, called Somatotypes are identified by certain physical characteristics. To determine your somatotype, please complete the following:

Name: _____

Address: _____

City, State Zip: _____

Age____ Sex ____ Phone ____-____-_____

For Office Use Only:

According to the attached questionnaire that you recently completed and returned to us, we have determined that you are the following somatotypes: _____.

Questionnaire

Answer the following questions as your body looks in its natural state without clothing. Circle each description, which relates to you then follow the instructions given in the box below:

☆ Thick muscles	☆ Chubby as a baby	☆ Small bones
☆ Solid muscle structure	☆ Chubby as adolescent	☆ Medium bones
☆ Long slim muscles	☆ Little body fat	☆ Rounded stomach
☆ Short neck	☆ Moderate body fat	☆ Large stomach
☆ Long, narrow hands and feet	☆ Heavy body fat	☆ Thin face
☆ Round face	☆ I lose weight easily	☆ Squared face
☆ Very strong	☆ I gain weight easily	☆ Have to lift weights to have any muscle
☆ Long arms and legs	☆ Large pecs	☆ Have muscle tone without weights
☆ Short arms and legs	☆ Large leg muscles	☆ I have to eat a lot to gain weight
☆ Short waisted	☆ Wide hips	☆ I have to watch my diet or I gain body fat
☆ Long waisted	☆ Narrow hips	
☆ Flat stomach	☆ Medium hips	
☆ Large chest	☆ Large bones	

☆ My weight stays about the   same no matter what I eat

       Please complete the above questionnaire and return it to The Complete Health System, 646 South Main Street, Lock Box 304, Cedar City, UT 84720 along with $9.95 made payable to Applied Web Info Please include a self-addressed stamped envelope (SASE). Also, please allow ten (10) days for delivery of your answered questionnaire. All questionnaires submitted without an SASE and the proper processing fee will not be processed. All questionnaires are confidential.

Chapter 10: Healthy Facts for Healthy Living

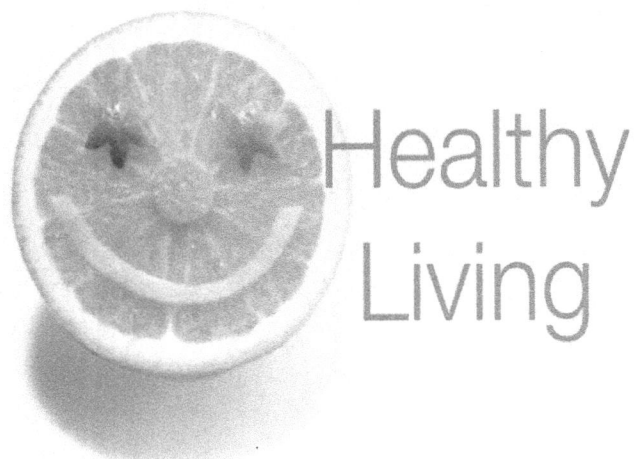

☆ Using apple cider vinegar for athlete's foot and jock itch. Simply spray it on or rub it on and wait until dry. When dry, vinegar has the same "ph" level as your skin so it is odorless. Be careful not to get it on your clothes or you'll smell like a Caesar's salad.

☆ Put vinegar in your dishwasher and buy the least expensive dishwasher soap. Vinegar is a great grease cutter and dries spot free.

☆ Use lemon juice to make your fingernails whiter. The lemon juice actually bleaches them white.

☆ Crawling insects hate the smell of bay leaves. Place them in your drawers and cupboards.

☆ Basil plants repel insects and flies. Place them in your house and enclosed patio.

☆ Rats and mice hate steel wool. Use it to stuff into holes and crevasses that they can enter through.

☆ Use tin foil around your plants to keep most animals away from them.

☆ Mice hate the smell of peppermint. Place oil of peppermint on a rag and put it in your cupboards.

☆ Ants hate the smell of whole cloves, cucumber peelings and Ivory Liquid Soap.

☆ To unclog a drain, use vinegar and baking soda and then stand back for some quick action.

☆ Baking soda added to dishwater cuts grease on dishes and is very inexpensive.

☆ By placing an ice cube overnight on carpet that has been matted down by furniture, it will cause it to be back up by morning.

- Flat club soda is excellent for plants.

- Warm vinegar will remove most decals. Allow it to soak in for a few minutes.

- To take the dents out of ping-pong balls, place them in hot water for 15-20 minutes.

- For a smoother texture and longer life, nail polish should be stored in the refrigerator.

- Pantyhose will last longer if you freeze them before wearing.

- Eating a piece of bacon that does not taste salty is an indication that you are eating too much salt.

- If you get migraine headaches, avoid aged wine and cheeses.

- If you want clear ice cubes, boil the water first.

- To make your hair shiny, try adding a teaspoon of vinegar in your final rinse.

- Vinegar makes a great rust and mildew remover from chrome.

- Use old milk cartons for large ice cubes. The bigger the cube, the slower it melts.

- Apple seeds, plum pits and apricot pits are the most dangerous toxic fruit seeds.

- There are 110 pesticides used on apples alone.

- Pectin, found in most citrus fruits, is effective in lowering cholesterol.

- In a recent study, the chemical called solanine was found effective against arthritis pain. Foods containing solanine are green potatoes, tomatoes, red and green peppers, eggplant and paprika.

- Parsley is effective in overcoming bad breath.

- The sugar content found in most beans cause intestinal gas.

- Soybeans and broccoli are the most nutritious vegetables.

- To determine if a mushroom is safe or poisonous, sprinkle salt on the gills. If it turns yellow, it is poisonous; if it turns black it is safe.

- If you chew gum while peeling onions, you will not cry.

- If you hate the taste of vitamins, store them in the refrigerator but never freeze them. Freezing them crystallizes some of the nutrients rendering them inert.

- PMS robs the body of vitamin C.

- Breast cancer rates are highest in areas with the least amount of sunshine. Lack of vitamin D could be the problem.

- Beta Carotene is only available from plants. Vitamin A comes from animal sources.

- Never take vitamin C and aspirin together. Studies indicate that when combined, heavy doses produce excessive stomach irritation, which may lead to ulcers.

☆ The lowest quality meat and poultry is used in canned goods, frozen foods and TV dinners.

☆ Depleted soils are the result of farming only using fertilizers that only replace minerals crucial to crop growth such as phosphorous, potassium and nitrates.

☆ Smokers require 40% more vitamin C.

☆ Eating foods high in fat makes you full longer. Approximately 10 grams of fat is cleared from the stomach per hour. Two eggs, bread and butter, coffee and milk equals 50 grams of fat. Assimilation takes 5-6 hours.

☆ One pound of charcoal barbecued meat contains as much carcinogens as the smoke of 15 cigarettes.

☆ The average person consumes 129 gallons of fluid per year. For optimum health, 64 ounces (1-gallon) of pure water should be consumed each day for total water consumption alone of 365 gallons per year.

☆ The colder the water we drink with our meals, the slower the digestive process.

☆ It takes 5-gallons of water to produce 1-gallon of milk, 100,000-gallons of water to produce one car and 280-gallons of water to print 1-copy of the Sunday newspaper.

☆ 47% of our nation's water supply goes for food production.

☆ 2/3 of all US households are drinking water that violates EPA standards.

☆ Americans spend over $2-Billion/year on bottled water and almost the same amount on filtration and purification systems.

☆ 70% of Americans are concerned about the quality of their drinking water.

☆ In a 24-hour period, 55-tons of caffeine and 985-tons of alcohol are consumed in the US.

☆ Approximately $50 Million worth of Twinkies were sold in the US in 1990.

☆ Americans drink 4,848 cups of coffee every second of every day.

☆ The average American consumes 1800 pounds of food per year.

☆ Food manufacturers spend $4 Billion for advertising each year.

☆ Over a billion pounds of chemical additives are consumed every year.

☆ White bread may have as many as 16 chemical additives just to keep it fresh!

☆ When grocery shopping, the highest profit items are placed at eye level.

☆ Check the bottom of lettuce. If the ring is brown, do not buy it. It should be white.

☆ Foods on the lowest shelves are usually the least expensive.

☆ The most commonly purchased items are usually found in the center of an aisle.

☆ In one year, the average American consumes 100 lbs. of refined sugar, 55 lbs. of fats and oils, 300 cans of soft drinks, 200 sticks of gum, 18 lbs. of candy, 5 lbs. of potato chips, 7 lbs. of popcorn, 63 dozen doughnuts, 50 lbs. of cakes and cookies, 20 gallons of ice cream, 209 lbs. of vegetables, and 149 lbs. of fruit.

☆ Americans eat approximately 6 pounds of chemical additives per year. The liver is the major organ that has the job of breaking down and disposing of all this material. If certain nutrients necessary to break them down are not available, problems will occur.

☆ Pasta products are considered a low-fat food and are easily digested due to their low fiber content. Perfect for babies!

☆ Having trouble estimating pasta amounts? Remember this: one cup of uncooked pasta equals two cups of cooked pasta.

☆ To obtain the right amount of water to cook rice without measuring, place the uncooked rice in the pan and shake it to level it. Add water until it is one inch above the level rice.

☆ Decaffeinated coffee is the most harmful to you due to the chemical process used to decaffeinate the beans. If you use decaf, buy only the brands that use the "water" process, preferably the "Swiss Process". Also, brewed coffee is good for you if you use the unbleached brown coffee filters instead of the white filters. White filters contain dioxin. Instant coffee is the best and has 50% less caffeine than brewed coffee.

Chapter 11: Cholesterol (Current research)

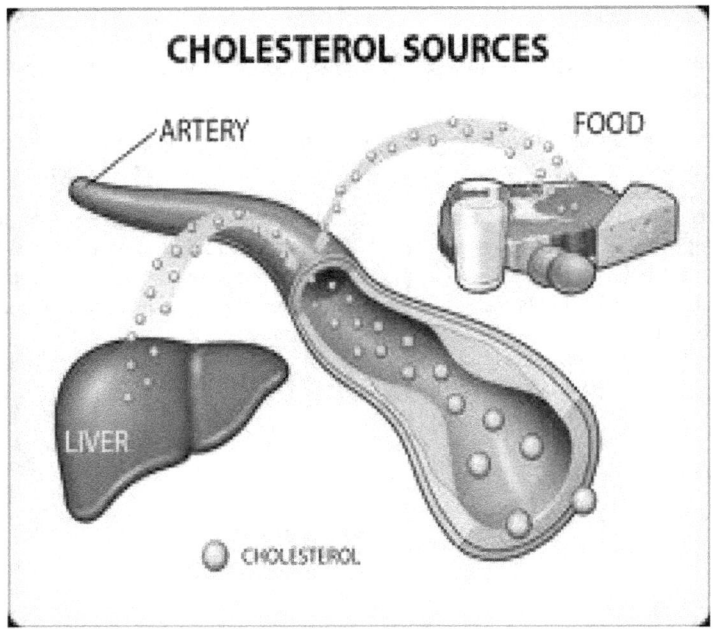

CHOLESTEROL SOURCES

ARTERY

FOOD

LIVER

CHOLESTEROL

The word itself evokes images of arteries narrowed by atherosclerotic plaque, the gunk that sticks to vessels and impedes the passage of blood the way a kink in a garden hose slows the flow of water. Or perhaps we think of cholesterol as something our favorite foods—ice cream, two-crust pies, steaks, French fries—are rich in, a culinary spoiler that makes us choose the fish yet again. (Hold the Béarnaise, please.) But the drumbeat of public health messages about the hazards of too much dietary cholesterol obscures a more complex reality, namely that cholesterol is essential to animal life. In fact, much of the cholesterol in us is manufactured by our own bodies, not obtained from our foods. It serves as a precursor to the sex hormones estradiol and testosterone and to vitamin D, which is necessary for the formation of bone. Cholesterol is also needed to produce the bile acids that digest fats. Cholesterol is only dangerous when the body's regulation of it goes awry, owing to genetic or environmental causes.

The most fascinating aspect of cholesterol is its role in regulating membrane fluidity in animal cells. Far from being simple walls, cell membranes are instead complicated liquid crystals. About 50 percent of a cell membrane is composed of lipids (oily organic compounds like fats) and most of the rest is made of proteins. The whole lot is characterized by randomness, chaos, and subtlety. Membranes are not rigid little sheets. They fluctuate, they're dynamical systems, and they are remarkable. The normal fluidity of cell membranes is now thought essential to life functions, and disruptions can have dire consequences. Just this year scientists reported that cholesterol's regulation of membrane fluidity may be involved in the destruction of brain cells that leads to Alzheimer's disease; that reduced fluidity in the membranes of red blood cells may be related to psoriasis outbreaks; that abnormalities in membrane lipid content may cause resistance to leptin, the hormone that regulates appetite to maintain normal body weight; and that chromium, a carcinogen, causes tumors by reducing membrane fluidity. Membrane fluidity is probably involved in all cell processes associated with communication of cells with each other and with the outside world. Experimental studies suggest that membrane fluidity and cellular communication are related.

Membranes consisting of the lipid diphenoylphosphatidylcholine and cholesterol undergo a clear phase transition between a gel and a fluid state at a lipid/cholesterol ratio of about eight. At this and higher concentrations of cholesterol, the lipid is held in a gel-like state by the cholesterol. At lower concentrations of cholesterol, the lipid melts into a fluid state. This observation is significant, because phase change is associated with a significant change in the character of the cell membrane. **The high-cholesterol gel phase is much less fluid than the low-cholesterol phase.** The cholesterol-induced phase change observed in a membrane patch in the computer shows the mechanism for the experimentally observed cholesterol-induced fluidity changes, presumably those associated with the normal processes of cell fusion and perhaps even the pathology of Alzheimer's disease.

Another study looks at the ion channel proteins embedded in cell membranes. These little living batteries convert the chemical potential of ions into electrical currents. They are essential to intercellular signaling and to transporting material between the inside and the outside of a cell. If scientists can understand these biomolecules on the atomic level—understand exactly how a given protein structure results in an observed current—then it should be possible to engineer ion channels into the workhorses of nanodevices built partly of biological materials.

Eventually the components of highly sophisticated nanodevices might be embedded into such engineered cell membranes. Such nanodevices would live in the body much like any other cell, taking over functions lost to disease or injury. Although scientists have already demonstrated the feasibility of building such hybrid nanodevices, much more work is needed before such devices can be successfully installed and function in a living organism.

Chapter 12: Natural Treatment Protocols

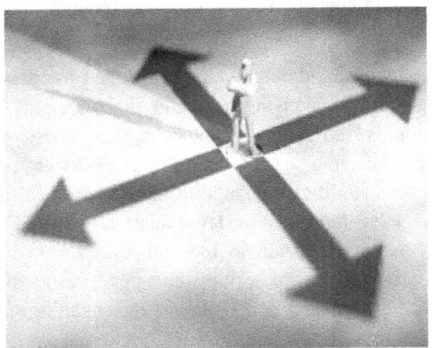

The following is a list of 151 natural, home remedies for everyday injuries, diseases, and ailments. All of the ingredients for the remedies are natural, and are available in most health food stores, and even some major supermarket chains. Many ingredients can also be grown at home, or are household products. These remedies, however, are not replacements for traditional medicine; they are just time and money saving alternatives. If there is a medical emergency, or symptoms persist for an excessive amount of time, please consult a doctor or go to the emergency room. The best medicine, however, is preventive medicine, so eat healthy, exercise, and take care of yourself before an illness takes hold.

1. Abscess / Boils
2. Abrasions (cuts, wounds)
3. Aches
4. Acne
5. Afterbirth / Pain
6. Age Spots
7. Allergies
8. Anemia
9. Appetite
10. Arteriosclerosis
11. Arthritis

12. Asthma
13. Athlete's Foot
14. Back Care
15. Bad Breath
16. Balding
17. Bedsores
18. Bedwetting
19. Birth Defects
20. Bites / Stings
21. Bladder Problems
22. Bleeding / Hemorrhage
23. Blisters
24. Blood Pressure
25. Body Odor
26. Bone Knitting
27. Brain Care
28. Breast Care
29. Bronchitis
30. Bruises
31. Bursitis
32. Burns
33. Cancer / Tumors
34. Chicken Pox
35. Choking
36. Childbirth
37. Circulation
38. Cleansing (Colon)
39. Colic
40. Colds
41. Colitis
42. Constipation
43. Convulsions
44. Corns

45. Cough

46. Cradle Cap

47. Cramps

48. Croup

49. Dandruff

50. Dermatitis

51. Diabetes

52. Diaper Rash

53. Diarrhea

54. Dislocations

55. Dizziness

56. Dry Skin

57. Ear Infections

58. Eczema

59. Emphysema

60. Lack of Energy

61. Eye Care

62. Facial Care

63. Fever

64. Fingernails

65. Foot Care

66. Frostbite

67. Gas

68. Gout

69. Hair Care / Loss

70. Headaches

71. Heartburn

72. Heart Care

73. Hemorrhoids

74. Hepatitis

75. Hernia / Rupture

76. Hearing Loss

77. Herpes

78. Hiccups
79. Hives
80. Laryngitis
81. Hyperactivity
82. Hypoglycemia
83. Indigestion
84. Inflammation
85. Insomnia
86. Itching
87. Lactation
88. Leg Pains
89. Liver Care
90. Lumbago
91. Lungs
92. Lupus
93. Lymph Glands
94. Measles
95. Memory
96. Menopause
97. Menstruation
98. Migraines
99. Miscarriages
100. Morn Sickness
101. Motion Sickness
102. Mouth Sores
103. Mucus / Congestion
104. Mumps
105. Nausea
106. Nerves
107. Nightmares
108. Nosebleed
109. Osteoporosis
110. Pain

Abscess / Boils

Apply cayenne extract, wintergreen oil, or a strong comfrey root tea to the boil or abscess. This will help bring the stigma to a head as well as aid the drying and mending process. Use these herbs or extract form: Mix one part lobelia with three parts mullein in a little warm water. Soak a clean cloth into the mixture and apply it to the sore to bring it to a head. Then puncture the wound lightly with a sterile needle. Wash gently. Apply garlic oil to prevent infection. When the redness has subsided apply vitamin E oil twice daily to aid healing. Drink comfrey root tea to speed healing action. Lecithin, zinc, and B-complex supplements taken daily will help prevent and remedy such sores.

Abrasions (cuts, wounds)

Apply aloe vera gel, vitamin E oil, or cod liver oil to the washed wound. To reduce infection and inflammation put garlic oil on a band-aid and cover the wound. Sprinkle cayenne pepper on a small clean cut to stop the bleeding and knit the wound.

Aches

Apply lobelia or cayenne extract to the painful area to relax muscles and hasten healing. Apply moist heat directly to an ache and rest. Take the herbs lobelia or valerian root in capsules to relax the muscles and to ease the pain. Take B-complex, calcium, and cayenne supplements to heal muscles and to prevent recurring aches.

Acne

Gently scrub acne with a mixture of chickweed herb and water to reduce inflammation. Apply garlic oil and cayenne extract, or a Redmond clay poultice, to draw out toxins and to heal the acne. Avoid eating chocolate, fried food, and refined sugar. Take B-complex and zinc supplements daily to strengthen the skin's resistance to acne. The herbs cayenne, garlic, ginseng, burdock, and sarsaparilla taken orally can help rid the skin of blemishes. Avoid over washing the skin, this dries out the skin and irritates it.

Afterbirth / Pain

Make a strong tea of the herbs red raspberry, St.-John's-wort, valerian root, or wild yam. Drink this after labor to reduce pain. Nutmeg tea will help to contract the uterus and to lessen bleeding. Take the herbs cayenne, yarrow, mistletoe, or corn silk in capsules to reduce bleeding. Both chlorophyll and the herb shepherd's-purse are rich in vitamin K. This makes them helpful in the clotting of blood.

Age Spots

Apply vitamin E oil or cod liver oil directly to age spots everyday to reduce coloration. Selenium and the herbs dandelion, ginseng, gotu kola, licorice, and sarsaparilla may prove helpful taken in capsules or drunk as teas. Take 4,000 mgs of good quality flaxseed oil in gel caps daily.

Allergies

Make a tea of the herb goldenseal or eyebright. Strain; put the cooled tea in a dropper bottle. Use this as an eyewash to reduce the burning, watering, and the inflammation caused by many allergies. To build up resistance to allergies, diet is important. Avoid dairy products, sugar, and refined foods. Take vitamin C, pantothenic acid, and dolomite supplements. Parsley and bee pollen decrease allergic reactions. Take the herbs juniper and comfrey in capsules for prevention. Take cayenne pepper and garlic together to dry up the sinuses.

Appetite

A thiamine deficiency is often the cause of a loss of appetite. Take a thiamine supplement along with B-complex, vitamin A, zinc, niacin, and biotin. These work well together and help in the assimilation of the thiamine. Drink peppermint tea to help increase the appetite. Take the herb fennel in capsules to normalize the appetite. Any combination of the following will increase the appetite: barberry, garlic, ginseng, goldenseal, hops, horseradish, oat straw, parsley, and safflower. The herb chickweed will decrease one's appetite.

Arteriosclerosis

A beneficial healing herbal combination is garlic, cayenne, and hawthorn. Garlic cleanses cholesterol from the bloodstream making deposits less sticky. Hawthorn regulates the blood pressure and strengthens the nerves to the heart making the heart stronger. Cayenne pepper helps to cleanse the circulatory system, strengthen the pulse rate and regulate the heart and blood pressure. Cayenne will also increase the effectiveness of other herbs. Vitamin C helps to prevent blood clots and fatty deposits in the arteries. Lecithin will break up cholesterol and carry it away. Magnesium and calcium protect against fatty deposits. Stick to whole foods and a low fat diet. Avoid white flour products, sugar laden, and oily foods. Garlic, onions, and eggplant have the wonderful ability to balance the cholesterol level. Pectin, in apples, helps to prevent the absorption of cholesterol. A B-6 complex deficiency when you are pregnant can cause arteriosclerosis in the infant.

Arthritis

To relieve pain and help in the healing process, apply one of these to the sore area: lobelia extract, cayenne extract, or halibut oil. Exercise moderately to ease stiffness. Much of the pain of arthritis is caused by a lack of minerals in one's diet. Take bone meal and dolomite supplements daily to get these minerals. The herb oat straw will help the body use the minerals. Alfalfa is very rich in minerals and vitamins. Drink alfalfa tea and take supplements. Parsley is high in nutrients, and would be a wise addition to one's diet. Be sure your daily vitamin supplement contains B-6, vitamin C, vitamin E, magnesium, and niacin. These will help prevent stiffness. The herbs yucca and burdock will help reduce inflammation and swelling. To ensure that you are getting plenty of the needed nutrients, add these foods to your diet: pecans, bananas, brewer's yeast, wheat germ, avocados, cherries, and green salads.

Asthma

Bee pollen is quite nutritionally rich; taking it daily will gradually chase away those allergens. Take cayenne and garlic to heal, comfort, and help build a strong constitution. Ginseng should be taken to help the body improve its capacity to resist and endure. It will also

69

assist the endocrine glands in the assimilation of vitamins and minerals. Take plenty of vitamins A, D, and B-complex, PABA and pantothenic acid. Avoid dairy products, which contribute to phlegm build-up. Take lobelia extract to lessen the severity of asthma attacks.

Athlete's Foot

Rub the affected area with white vinegar. Apply brewer's yeast and honey twice daily. Dust feet with cornstarch before putting on shoes or socks. Avoid plastic or vinyl shoes. Vinegar has the same ph level, as your skin when it has dried hence there is no odor.

Back Care

Rub lobelia extract on sore muscles. Lobelia is a strong muscle relaxant. Prepare a strong comfrey tea and drink to reduce a swollen back. Take the herbs lobelia or valerian root with cayenne to relax the muscles, to help you rest, to relieve the pain, and to heal the injured area.

Bad Breath

Brush the teeth well and floss regularly. Cleanse the colon. Bad breath is often caused by toxins stored in the large intestine. To cover odor, eat parsley, drink peppermint tea, chew cloves, take chlorophyll, or gargle with barberry tea. Take acidophilus or chew uemboshi plums to improve intestinal flora. To insure proper digestion, chew food well, and drink water in between meals. Calcium, B-complex and C vitamins and the herb myrrh can prevent bad breath when taken daily.

Balding

Shampoo with a tea made from yarrow herb to open the pores and encourage hair growth. Drink yarrow to reduce balding. Take copper, insitol, vitamin B-complex, and vitamins C and E. Take the herb sage to encourage hair growth. Eat wakeme and hijiki seaweed to prevent balding.

Bed Sores

Apply pure honey, liquid lecithin, or zinc ointment to a clean sore. Dress it with a gauze bandage. Take vitamin C, A, and B-complex, as well as folic acid and zinc.

Bedwetting

Take the herbs corn silk and ursi to prevent bed-wetting. Eat parsley or chew on cinnamon bark. Avoid sugary foods, chocolate, meat, fruit, or artificial additives.

Birth Defects

To improve the health of the reproductive system during pregnancy, drink red raspberry tea. Alfalfa, dandelion, and kelp prevent birth defects by providing a rich source of iron and iodine. Take extra vitamin E while pregnant to heal the reproductive organs. Avoid cigarette smoke, alcohol, sugar, drugs, and caffeine while pregnant. Alcohol is the leading cause of retardation in newborn babies.

Bites / Stings

Apply one of the following to bites or stings to reduce pain and swelling: aloe vera gel, garlic oil, baking soda and water, vinegar, honey, plaintain tea, or safflower oil. Use lemon juice and cornstarch or lobelia extract and myrrh to relieve persistent pain and itch. Pennyroyal tea mixed with a drop of eucalyptus oil can be applied to the skin as an insect repellant. Dried tomato leaves can keep bugs out of your house when hung by windows. Taking garlic supplements, or eating garlic, will lessen your chances of bug bites (and vampire bites).

Bladder / Kidney Problems

Take psyllium husk and water daily to cleanse the colon. A colon full of toxins puts pressure on the bladder and leads to infection. Avoid packaged douches, tight nylons or underwear, or satin underwear. Urinate before and after sexual intercourse. To cleanse the bladder and kidneys of excess mucus and irritants, take the herbs St.-John's-wort or alfalfa in capsule form. Drink dandelion and peach bark tea. Take garlic and goldenseal in addition to vitamin C to fight infection. Take dolomite and water to fight bladder infections. Eat whole fresh cranberries to cleanse the kidneys. The herbs blessed thistle and white oak bark work well together in capsules or as teas toward healing infection. Drink dolomite with water to heal bladder infections. Grind fresh cranberries in the blender and add to plain yogurt (or soy yogurt) and eat daily. The herbs buchu and ura ursi rid the bladder of excess mucus, infection, gravel, stones, and retained water.

Bleeding / Hemorrhage

Apply cayenne extract or powder to a small wound to stop the bleeding. Make a strong tea of one of the following: slippery elm, plantain, white oak bark,

72

comfrey, nettle, or chaparral. Apply the tea directly to the wound to stop bleeding. Capsules of cayenne, bistort, goldenseal, and white oak bark, yarrow, or comfrey can stop internal bleeding. The herb don quai, in capsule form, can break up blood clots. Consult a doctor if there is: Bleeding from the rectum, lungs, stomach, or uterus. Blood in the urine. Large wounds with uncontrollable bleeding. Blood in the vomit or mucus from a cough.

Blisters

Apply vitamin E oil or zinc ointment or aloe vera gel twice daily. Apply garlic oil to infected blisters.

Blood Pressure

High blood pressure results in part from a sodium-potassium imbalance caused by too much salt consumption. Bananas and whole wheat bread are rich in potassium to balance sodium levels. Stay away from salt, sugar, dairy products, processed food, and meats. Take valerian root to relax. Take dolomite in water. Exercise daily. Cayenne, garlic, and the herb passionflower regulate both high and low blood pressure. Ginseng, hyssop, and hawthorn, taken together, regulate high and low blood pressure. The herb barberry dilates the blood vessels and helps to bring high blood pressure down. Vitamin E and zinc, taken daily, will help reduce high blood pressure.

Body Odor / Perspiration

Apply baking soda to clean armpits and feet to reduce odor. Soak feet in warm water and horsetail herb tea. Cleanse the colon with chlorophyll enemas to rinse out toxins. Toxins in the colon spread odors throughout

73

the body. The herb yarrow will open pores and result in more perspiration.

Bone Knitting

Apply comfrey tea poultice to a bone fracture or break, also drink comfrey tea often. Take dolomite and bone meal supplements to build bones. Valerian root and cayenne pepper, taken with vitamin C, will dull the pain and help to heal the bones. Serious breaks should be treated by a doctor, and put into a cast.

Brain Care

Optimal brain function is aided by a whole foods diet rich in protein, and avoids sugar, caffeine, additives, and preservatives. Take vitamin C, E, and B-complex. The herbs gotu kola and ginseng help to strengthen the memory.

Breast Care

Apply one of the following to sore, inflamed nipples: cod liver oil, white oak bark tea, vitamin E oil, garlic oil, or parsley leaves that have been steeped in white vinegar for five minutes. Refer to the Women's Health section for instructions on how to perform a monthly breast exam. Drink red raspberry tea to keep the breasts healthy.

Bronchitis

Rub the throat and chest with garlic oil or cayenne extract to loosen congestion and lessen coughs. Take garlic, cayenne, and ginger together to clean and heal the bronchial tubes. An herbal mix of lobelia, eucalyptus, and comfrey will relax the system, loosen congestion, and

74

reduce coughing. Mullein or peppermint tea lessens the severity of the symptoms. Capsules of juniper berries will dilate the bronchial tubes and reduce inflammation.

Bruises

Apply cold water or ice to bruises to reduce initial swelling. Steep mullein flowers in olive oil and apply to bruises as an ointment. Apply a tea of: comfrey, hops, hyssop, white oak bark, or St.-John's-wort. Take lobelia and comfrey in capsules to help heal a bruise. To prevent from bruising easily, take a bioflavanoid supplement.

Bursitis

Apply ice to the injured area to relieve pain and inflammation. Soak a cloth in strong comfrey or mullein tea and apply often to the injured area. Apply lobelia extract to the joint to prevent stiffness, crippling, and to relax the joint and ease the pain. Drink an herbal tea of chamomile, hops, and skullcap to speed the healing process. Cayenne and lobelia taken in capsules will help to heal and reduce inflammation. The herbal mixture of alfalfa, comfrey, and chaparral decreases soreness and soothes inflammation.

Burns

Immediately apply cold water cloths to burns to prevent further tissue damage. Throughout the first day, continually apply aloe vera gel or cucumber juice. Treat the burn with vitamin E; cod liver oil, honey, plain yogurt, or a strong, cold herbal tea of plantain, comfrey, burdock, or pennyroyal. Apply garlic oil to an infected burn. If skin is broken, soak a clean cloth in red raspberry or slippery elm tea and apply to the burn. Drink aloe vera juice to hasten healing. Avoid lanolin lotions, because lanolin intensifies a burn. See a doctor if you have serious or extensive burns.

Cancer / Tumors

The following herbal teas may be applied topically to reduce swelling: pokeweed, mullein, and lobelia, or plantain and horseradish. The herbs pokeweed, red clover, chaparral, and yellow dock may be taken together in capsules to purify the blood and break up tumors or growths. Take the herb taheebo to dull the pain. Drink a strong tansy tea to soothe symptoms and promote healing. To prevent certain cancers, abstain from eating meat products, smoking, and alcohol.

Chicken Pox

A warm bath with one of the following herbs in it: ginger, goldenseal, burdock, or yellow dock will soothe itching and rash. Apply garlic oil, vitamin E oil, or liver oil to sores. To relieve a fever, take either cayenne or lobelia extract in water. Take garlic capsules to fight infection. Drink saffron and snake root tea to lessen the severity of the symptoms.

Choking

A person is choking when food lodges in the throat and no air can pass through. A choking person can't cough or talk. To dislodge food or an object from the throat, place your fist above the victim's navel and below the rib cage. Push up forcefully with an upward thrust. Repeat if necessary.

Childbirth

Drinking raspberry tea during pregnancy strengthens the uterus, which will coordinate contractions and shorten labor. Take the herbs cramp bark and wild yam together to relieve leg pains and to prevent miscarriages. The herb corn silk can bring about labor and reduce bleeding after labor. Nutmeg tea helps the uterus to contract and lessens afterbirth bleeding. Take the herb thyme in a tea to help expel the placenta. Apply myrrh to the newborn's navel after the cord has been removed to prevent infection. Take St.-John's-wort in capsules to relieve afterpain. The herbs pennyroyal and mistletoe may induce abortion by causing uterine contractions and miscarriage.

Circulation

Massage the body with cayenne extract to improve circulation. Sprinkle powdered cayenne pepper into socks and gloves to keep the feet and hands warm. Take vitamins C and E to improve circulation. After bathing, give the body a vigorous massage with a terrycloth towel.

Cleansing (Colon)

Take psyllium seed with lots of water at night to cleanse the colon of mucus, toxins, stored wastes, and parasites. Take acidophilus in capsule form to control harmful bacteria and to prevent gas, bad breath, bloating, and constipation. Drink lots of water to cleanse the system. Add 3 T. of ginger root to a warm bath to open the pores and rid the body of toxins.

Colic

Rub lobelia extract or hops tea on the baby's spine to relax it. Give the baby a mild tea of peppermint, catnip, fennel, or hops. The lack of vitamin B6 may promote colic in a baby. To get vitamin B6, feed the baby creamed brown rice or brewer's yeast in applesauce. Sugar worsens the colic symptoms. Feed the baby no sugar, and if breast-feeding, the mother should also avoid sugar.

Colds

Sniff peppermint oil vapor to open sinuses. Rub cayenne, garlic oil and lobelia onto the throat for relief from coughs, congestion, or sore throats. Take large amount of vitamin C. Vitamin C prevents viruses and bacteria from reproducing and also neutralizes harmful bacteria by reducing mucus in the cells. Take Co-enzyme Q10 to aid the effects of vitamin C. Garlic, cayenne, and goldenseal act as natural antibiotics and fight infection and reduce fever. Alfalfa halts sneezing attacks and clears sinuses. The herb fenugreek in capsules eases sinus headaches. The herb comfrey in tea or capsules soothes upset stomachs. Honey and lemon juice soothe sore throats and ease coughs. Dairy products cause excess mucus build-up, and should be avoided during a cold.

Colitis

Take papaya or peppermint with garlic or goldenseal to stimulate digestion and relieve inflammation. The herbs myrrh, slippery elm, and white oak bark taken separately will soothe and heal an inflamed intestine. Psyllium and water will cleanse the colon and relieve constipation. Take vitamins A, E, K,

78

and B-complex to hasten the healing process. The consumption of white flour products is a major contributor to the symptoms of colitis. Avoid bleached flour and refined foods.

Constipation

Exercise daily, especially brisk walking or jogging. Take the herbs psyllium, slippery elm, or fenugreek in capsules to lubricate, cleanse, and heal the colon. The herb cascara sagrada will relax, soothe, and strengthen the bowel tone. The following herbs are mild stool softeners and laxatives and may be taken individually or in combination: red clover, turkey rhubarb, comfrey, and don quai. Licorice and dandelion teas may be given to constipated babies or children. Take cayenne pepper in capsules to relieve bleeding hemorrhoids. Liquid chlorophyll helps to keep the bowels functioning properly. Drink aloe vera juice to improve intestinal flora and to alleviate constipation. Acidophilus capsules comfort spastic colons and promote healthy intestinal flora. Eat plenty of fiber and whole-wheat products with plenty of water to prevent constipation. Dried fruits like prunes, raisins, and dates are high fiber snacks.

Corns

Prepare a strong chamomile tea. Apply it to the corn frequently and cover with gauze to keep it clean.

Cough

Rub the throat with eucalyptus oil, lobelia extract, garlic oil, or a natural vapor rub. This will help expel mucus, relax the body, and reduce inflammation of the throat. Gargle with a strong tea made from sage leaves and elder blossoms. Add a drop of almond oil, oil of clove and some honey. This soothes the throat and lessens the severity of the cough. Inhale the steam from a strong coltsfoot tea. Drink the tea with honey and lemon to further soothe the throat. The herbs garlic, lobelia, comfrey and licorice work well together to combat coughing. A strong tea, made of red raspberry, honey suckle, or licorice, with honey also soothes the throat. Make a cough syrup out of the juice of a baked onion, strong comfrey tea, and honey. Take as needed.

Cradle Cap

Apply vitamin E or cod liver oil to the dry, flaky, scalp. Brush lightly with a soft bristled brush. Give the baby a drop of cod liver oil in some milk daily.

Cramps

Massage lobelia extract into any area that is cramped. Drink a tea of red raspberry leaves to prevent and reduce the severity of menstrual cramps. Take the herb hops in capsules or drink as a tea to calm the entire system. Drink a tea of comfrey leaves and alfalfa to lessen the pain of muscle cramps. Chamomile and peppermint tea relieve stomach cramps. Dolomite and vitamin E can help arm and leg cramps.

Croup

During an attack, turn on the shower to hot, and place the child in the steam filled room, until the coughing subsides. The steam helps to loosen phlegm and congestion and aid in free breathing. Put lobelia extract on the child's throat, chest, and back to relax the muscles.

Apply a cold cloth to the throat to reduce swelling. To reduce coughing, inflammation, and pain, drink, lobelia extract in water. Drink lemon juice and honey to soothe the throat.

Dandruff

Apply a strong tea of yarrow and chaparral to the scalp, and also drink the tea. Mix 3 T. of vinegar in one cup of water and rinse the hair with it. This removes shampoo residues that cause scalp irritation. Apply a tea of warm water, sage and rosemary to the scalp. Brush cornmeal through the hair to reduce excess oil. Take B6 and PABA to prevent dandruff.

Dermatitis

Apply aloe vera gel; cod liver oil, or vitamin E oil to the affected areas. Redmond clay, yellow dock, red clover, chickweed, and dandelion taken in capsules help heal dermatitis.

Diabetes

Take extra potassium, and vitamins E, C, and B-complex, to help keep the blood sugar at a healthy level. The herbs licorice, juniper, goldenseal, ura ursi, buchu, and cayenne may be taken in capsules to help heal diabetes. Take garlic pills to keep blood sugar levels down.

Diaper Rash

Apply garlic oil, aloe vera gel, vitamin E oil, lecithin, zinc ointment, cod liver oil, or mullein oil to the affected area. Give the baby a little cod liver orally twice a day to speed recovery.

Diarrhea

Drink red raspberry, slippery elm, comfrey, or clove tea, to lessen cramping, and to balance the bowel movements. The herbal tea mullein or slippery elm may be dilutes and used as enemas. Take acidophilus tablets and eat a teaspoon of nutmeg three times a day, to form a healthy stool. Eat carob and bananas to assist in balancing the stool's consistency.

Dislocations

Immediately apply a hot wet cloth to the injury for twenty minutes. Then pour cold water on the area to contract the muscle. Keep the bone in its proper position and consult a doctor. Take lobelia and cayenne to relax the muscles, ease the pain, and speed the healing process. Bone meal and dolomite help to strengthen the bones and prevent relapses.

Dizziness

Sit with the head between the knees to return the blood to the head. Use acupressure by squeezing the skin between the eyebrows with the thumb and index finger, Drink peppermint or chamomile tea to relax the system. Take a tablespoon of equal parts honey and apple cider vinegar twice daily to prevent dizzy spells.

Dry Skin

Apply cod liver oil, vitamin E oil, aloe vera gel, or honey to dry skin patches. Apply aloe vera gel after every shower or bath. Apply olive oil to a baby's dry skin. Take the herb don quai in capsules to moisten the skin. Take vitamins E and cod liver oil to make the skin soft and healthy.

82

Ear Infections / Aches

Drop garlic oil or lobelia extract into the ear and gently massage. Repeat four to five times a day. Apply ice to the ear to constrict the blood supply to the area and reduce the pain. Then apply a hot baked onion to the ear to reduce inflammation. Take lobelia extract in water to ease and relax the system. Take the herb hops in capsules or tea to heal an earache.

Eczema

Apply aloe vera gel; cod liver oil, or strawberry leaf tea to the irritated areas. Make a strong tea from comfrey, goldenseal, slippery elm, burdock and dandelion. Apply this to the skin four to six times a day. Take extra zinc, iron, and vitamins A, D, E, and B-complex to speed recovery. Drink aloe vera juice to cleanse the system. Avoid dairy products. They may cause or irritate eczema.

Emphysema

Rub the chest with garlic oil or eucalyptus oil to loosen phlegm. Drink a tea of garlic, rose hips, and fennel to ease coughing spells and promote healing. Take the herbs comfrey and fenugreek in capsules to loosen phlegm. The herbs marshmallow root, mullein, comfrey, chickweed, and slippery elm all work well together to ease the symptoms of emphysema.

Energy

The herbs licorice and cayenne in capsules act as a mild stimulant. The herbs ginseng, bee pollen, bayberry, dandelion, alfalfa, and brigham tea help to promote energy and vitality. The herb hawthorn taken with garlic or cayenne helps strengthen the heart. Avoid refined sugars that weaken the metabolism.

Eye Care

Place a slice of cucumber over each eye for relief from: irritation, and to get rid of dark circles under the eyes. Make a tea from any of these herbs: eyebright, goldenseal, witch hazel, or strawberry leaves. Use the cooled tea as an eyewash to reduce irritation. To reduce the swelling of a black eye, apply a cloth that has been soaked in hyssop or witch hazel tea. Apply vitamin E to wrinkles around the eyes, to reduce puffiness. The herbs fennel and eyebright taken in capsules strengthen the eyes and assist in fighting cataracts and glaucoma. Take cod liver oil and B-complex to strengthen the eyes.

Facial Care

Apply aloe vera gel to freshly washed skin to keep it moist and smooth. Prepare a facial of any one of the following: pure honey, oatmeal, plain yogurt, pureed strawberries, chamomile tea, wheat germ oil, or sunflower seed oil and water. Apply the mixture to face and leave on for fifteen minutes. Rinse with cold water. Use unscented facial products, and wash the face with aloe vera soaps.

Fever

Add 4 T. grated ginger to a warm bath. Soak in this to open the pores, and promote perspiration, to rid the body of toxins. Prepare a tea from parsley or red raspberry and drink often to bring the fever down. Also drink plenty of fluids. Take the combination of garlic and cayenne to promote healing and fight infection. Take

84

burdock, yarrow, goldenseal, dandelion, or Echinacea to reduce fever.

Fingernails

Apply vitamin E oil to split fingernails. Vitamin E, cod liver oil, iron, and dolomite taken internally help to build strong fingernails. The herbs horsetail, oat straw, comfrey, alfalfa, sage, and chamomile taken in capsules also help to strengthen nails.

Foot Care

Sprinkle cayenne pepper into socks to keep the feet warm. Rub baking powder onto the feet to avoid odors and keep the feet dry and clean. Take zinc supplements to fight foot odor. Drink strong horsetail tea to alleviate chronic foot odor.

Frostbite

Apply an ointment made by soaking mullein flowers in olive oil for fifteen minutes to the affected area. Repeat as needed. If the area becomes infected, apply garlic oil. Drink lobelia extract in water to lessen the pain. Eat fresh garlic, or garlic tablets to fight infection. See your doctor for serious cases of frostbite.

Gas

Take an enema of the herbal tea, catnip, for prompt gas relief. Eat dried papaya or drink papaya juice and peppermint tea to relieve gas pain. Take the following herbs, in combination, to alleviate stomach and colon gas: ginger, bayberry, wild yam, horseradish, ginseng, sage, psyllium, garlic, and safflower.

85

Gout

Apply a strong elm leaf tea to the painful area to relieve pain and inflammation. Take the herb safflower in capsules to heal gout. Drink unsweetened cherry juice to relieve the symptoms of gout. See "arthritis" Gout is a form of arthritis.

Hair Care / Loss

Occasionally cleanse the hair with white vinegar to rid it of shampoo and chemical residues. Rinse hair with a tea of yucca, sage, rosemary, or chamomile for added luster and shine. Apply pureed carrots to oily hair, pureed avocado to dry hair, or pureed cucumber to regular hair. Leave on for fifteen minutes and then rinse with cold water. Rinse the hair with peppermint or spearmint tea to improve circulation. Apply a mixture of raw egg and olive oil to the hair to prevent hair loss. Apply vitamin E oil or cod liver oil to dry, itchy scalp. Take PABA to control dandruff. Take pantothenic acid to thicken hair, repair split ends, and moisturize dry hair.

Headaches

Massage lobelia, cayenne, or valerian extract into the temples, forehead, neck, and shoulders. Drink a tea of peppermint and chamomile with lobelia extract to relax the head. Mix powdered wintergreen with white vinegar and drink it to relieve headaches fast. Wintergreen and vinegar is comparable to aspirin. Take the herb willow bark in capsules for relief. Willow bark contains salicin, which is the main component of aspirin. The following herbs also relieve headache pain: lobelia, valerian, cayenne, hops, wild lettuce, wood betony, thyme,

86

fenugreek, and ginger. The herb passionflower in capsules helps to relieve stress headaches.

Heartburn

Drink aloe vera juice, peppermint tea, or papaya juice. Papaya may also be taken in capsules to bring fast relief. The herbs cayenne, thyme, comfrey, and pepsin may also be taken to alleviate symptoms. Avoid fatty or fried foods, and exercise regularly.

Heart Care

See a doctor if you have the following symptoms: nausea, vomiting, and sweating, accompanied by a pain in the chest and the left shoulder and arm. Take dolomite to normalize cholesterol levels and to promote a healthy heart. The following herbs help to strengthen the heart and to cleanse the arteries and lower the blood pressure: hawthorn, garlic, and cayenne. Take lecithin, pectin, or alfalfa to lower the cholesterol level. Take the herb lobelia in small doses to control heart palpitations. The herb shepherd's-purse will slow heart palpitations if taken in small doses. Large doses may promote palpitations. Take small doses of the herb bayberry to excite the heart. Take large doses to slow the heart. Exercise regularly to strengthen the cardiovascular system.

Hemorrhoids

Directly apply cayenne extract or vitamin E oil to relieve itch and inflammation. Prepare a strong tea of witch hazel, slippery elm, goldenseal, or white oak bark and soak a clean cloth in it. Apply to the sore area. Chop up a cabbage and sit on it. This will soothe the hemorrhoids and the cabbage juice will draw toxins from the sores. Take cayenne pepper in capsules to relieve pain and bleeding. Drink witch hazel and comfrey tea to alleviate bleeding. Take the supplements rutin and bioflavanoids to prevent hemorrhoids. Take the herbs psyllium and turkey rhubarb with water to soften the stool.

Hepatitis

To help shake the symptoms, take the herbs barberry, cascara sagrada, and dandelion in capsules. Take a supplement of copper and sulfur.

Hernia / Rupture

Prepare a strong tea of the herb rupturewort. Soak a clean cloth in the tea and apply it to the injury. Take rupturewort in capsules to hasten healing. Take cayenne pepper in capsules to hasten healing.

Hearing Problems

Avoid using cotton swabs to clean the ears. They push against the eardrum and can cause damage to the membrane. They also push dirt further into the ear canal. Drop lobelia extract into the ear to relax the nerves. Use garlic oil to reduce inflammation. These will reduce ringing in the ears and will fight infection. Put a drop of glycerol into the ear to soften earwax so that it may fall out of the ear. Take lecithin and garlic supplements to fight ear infections.

Herpes Simplex

Apply vitamin E oil twice a day, to encourage the healing process. Vitamin E oil may also be taken in capsules to hasten healing. Take lysine supplements. This is a natural antibody that will destroy harmful bacteria and bring about a gradual healing of the disease. The herb taheebo may be taken in capsules to defend the body against disease by purifying the blood and by giving natural energy. Herpes sufferers should avoid peanuts and peanut products because they are rich in arginine, an amino acid that impedes the natural lysine in the body.

Hiccups

Drink lobelia extract in water to relax the throat and diaphragm. Drink a glass of water or orange juice without taking a breath. Hold your breath as long as possible.

Hives

Apply aloe vera gel or vitamin E oil twice daily. Take vitamin C, E, and zinc supplements every day. Take cayenne pepper in capsules to speed healing.

Hoarseness / Laryngitis

Rub the throat with lobelia extract. Prepare a strong tea of the herbs licorice, comfrey or hops. Drink or gargle. Take horseradish in capsules to soothe the larynx. Drink lobelia extract in capsules to soothe the throat.

Hyperactivity

Avoid chocolate, sugar, additives, aspirin, and artificial flavors and colors especially red dye. Stick to whole foods and low-sugar foods. Take extra B-complex and thiamine to help normalize the nervous system. Drop a little lobelia extract into water and drink to relax the system. Drink "near-beer" from health food stores, or any non-alcoholic beverage the contains hops, which helps in calming the system.

Hypoglycemia

Avoid alcohol, sweets, and caffeine. These cause headaches and other hypoglycemic symptoms. Eat frequent, small meals, and snack on nuts and seeds between mealtimes to maintain the blood sugar. The following herbs help to relieve hypoglycemic symptoms: licorice, juniper berries, garlic, dandelion, cayenne, alfalfa, kelp, hawthorn, and horse radish. Juniper berries help to strengthen the kidneys and adrenal glands, and assist in preventing hypoglycemia. Take valerian root to ease headache pain. Take calcium and vitamins B-complex, C, and E to promote endurance.

Indigestion

Drink aloe vera juice, papaya juice, or peppermint, chamomile, comfrey, or red raspberry tea to soothe the entire digestive tract. The following herbs taken in capsules will help heal the stomach: horse radish, papain, garlic, comfrey, thyme, wintergreen, cayenne, ginger, and red raspberry.

Inflammation

Apply garlic oil to the inflamed area. Cover with gauze to keep clean. Make a strong tea of comfrey or fenugreek. Soak a cloth in the tea and apply to the sore area. Apply a poultice of redmond clay to the wound. This will draw infection from the body. Take vitamin C to prevent bacteria from multiplying. Take garlic, myrrh, cayenne, goldenseal, or yucca to clear up an infection.

90

Insomnia

Sprinkle the herb basil in a warm bath and soak in it before bedtime to relax. Drink warm milk, chamomile, peppermint, or lobelia tea before bedtime to encourage sleepiness. The herbs hops, valerian, lobelia, skullcap, and passionflower may be taken together or separately to help relax the whole system and to calm the heart and nerves. Take iron, calcium, and potassium to encourage sleep.

Itching

Apply wheat germ oil, aloe vera gel, vitamin E oil, cod liver oil, witch hazel tea, or fresh lemon juice to the irritated area. Sprinkle the herbs yellow dock or peppermint into your bath water to reduce itching. Take the herbs plantain, yellow dock, chickweed, burdock, or goldenseal in capsules to eliminate annoying itch.

Lactation

Prepare a warm tea from the herb red raspberry or marshmallow root. Drink often to enrich and increase the flow of breast milk. The following herbs may be taken together or separately to improve the flow of milk as well as to enrich the milk: alfalfa, black walnut, fennel, horsetail, blessed thistle, comfrey, Irish moss, and oat straw. Papaya juice mixed with goat's milk makes an easily digested milk that can be used to wean an infant.

Leg Pains

Massage lobelia into the painful areas. Take cayenne and lobelia to heal. Take bone meal, dolomite, and vitamin E supplements to relieve persistent pain.

91

Liver Care

Avoid alcohol. Alcohol irritates the liver. Take the herbs dandelion and yellow dock to cleanse the liver and to purify the blood. The herb horseradish will help to reduce the size of a swollen liver. Drink strawberry leaf tea or peppermint tea to help heal liver ailments. For jaundice and cirrhosis, take vitamin E to aid with fat absorption. The herbs blessed thistle, cascara sagrada, garlic, fennel, safflower, barberry, catnip, and ginger may be taken in capsules to hasten the healing of liver ailments.

Lumbago

The herbs oat straw, comfrey, slippery elm, and valerian root work well together to combat the symptoms of lumbago. Take dolomite and vitamins E and B-complex to hasten healing.

Lungs

The herb pleurisy root helps heal all lung ailments. The herbs lobelia, thyme, and St.-John's-wort in capsules help the lungs to expel mucus. Chickweed, mullein, cayenne, bayberry, and yarrow are herbs that reduce bleeding in the lungs. The herbs marshmallow root, eucalyptus, and licorice may be taken in capsules together or separately to help heal and soothe the lungs. Drink comfrey or fenugreek tea to soothe the lungs.

Lupus

Take the supplements bone meal, dolomite, PABA, pantothenic acid, and vitamins A, C, D, and E. Consume foods that are rich in vitamin A, such as carrots, tomatoes, pink grapefruit, and red peppers.

Lymph Glands

Take the herbs myrrh and echinacea together in capsules to help cleanse the system and reduce glandular swelling.

Measles

Place equal portions of the herbs burdock, yellow dock, and goldenseal into a cheesecloth. Place this in a warm bath and soak in the brew to relieve irritated skin. Apply garlic oil to the affected areas to prevent infections. Soak in a warm bath of ginger and water to draw toxins from the body. Take garlic and valerian to fight infection and bring sleep. The herbs yarrow and lobelia in capsules help heal and relax the body. Drink saffron and snake root tea to speed the healing process.

Memory

Take the herbs ginseng and gotu kola together in capsules to prevent senility, improve the memory, and to promote mental endurance. B-complex, choline, and thiamine supplements will help normalize the nervous system and regulate nerve impulses to the brain. Avoid chocolate, sugar, alcohol, and smoking. These will irritate the entire nervous system.

Menopause / Hot Flashes

The following herbs taken in any combination will help to regulate the hormones that cause menopausal symptoms: damiana, life root, motherwort, black cohosh (natural estrogen) don quai, passionflower, sarsparilla, and ginseng. The herb valerian root may be taken in capsules to stop headaches and to promote sleepiness. Avoid caffeine, as this will aggravate the symptoms.

93

Menstruation

Take cayenne pepper in capsules to regulate the blood flow. The herb goldenseal taken with very small doses of mistletoe will reduce the blood flow. The herbs chamomile, parsley, squaw vine, and safflower will promote blood flow.

The following herbs alleviate the symptoms of cramps, leg, back, and headaches: hops, false unicorn, blessed thistle, and blue cohosh. Chlorophyll will help replace the calcium that is lost during menstruation.

Migraines

Daily supplements of dolomite and B-complex will assist in the prevention of migraines. A cup of chamomile tea everyday will also help prevent migraines. The following herbs help to ward off migraines: lobelia, fenugreek, thyme, wood betony, fennel, garlic, chamomile, cayenne, and blessed thistle. Valerian root, cayenne, and wild lettuce taken together will reduce the pain and assist in the healing.

Miscarriage

The herbs cramp bark and hawthorn may be taken in capsules to help prevent miscarriages. The herbs red raspberry, false unicorn, and lobelia help to strengthen the uterus, which will assist in shortening labor. Take them regularly during pregnancy. The herbs catnip and cayenne in capsules help to prevent morning sickness. The herbs bayberry and mistletoe help in stopping bleeding from the uterus.

Morning Sickness

A deficiency of calcium, B-complex, and B6 vitamins often cause nausea, which leads to vomiting. Drink a tea of red raspberry, peach leaf, alfalfa, peppermint, or ginger to help settle the stomach.

Motion Sickness

Tape a pickled umeboshi plum to the navel to prevent nausea. Begin taking vitamin B6 three days before your trip. Drink peppermint tea to calm the stomach.

Mouth Sores

Apply one of the following remedies to the sore: plain yogurt, aloe vera gel, garlic oil, liquid acidophilus culture, pure vanilla, or vitamin E oil. The powdered form of myrrh or white oak bark can be mixed with vitamin E oil and applied to very painful or persistent canker sores. Take plenty of acidophilus culture and avoiding acidic foods (like coffee and soda) will help prevent mouth sores. Mouth sores are also caused by an acidic stomach. To reduce inflammation and bleeding, rinse and gargle with one of the following: red raspberry, goldenseal, white oak bark, witch hazel, bistort, myrrh, comfrey, or wintergreen. Take zinc, B-complex, vitamin E, and bioflavanoids supplements to speed healing.

Mucus / Congestion

Apply cayenne extract or garlic oil to the chest to help relive congestion. Put peppermint or eucalyptus oil on a cloth and sniff it to help clear sinus congestion. Inhale the vapors of a tea of coltsfoot or mullein to open up the sinuses. Take garlic and cayenne in capsules to prevent congestion and to expel excess mucus. Take juniper berries in capsules to prevent excess mucus from forming. The herbs licorice or chickweed may be taken in teas or capsules to expel mucus from the respiratory tract. Yarrow clean mucus from the bladder, while St.-John's-wort cleans the bowels and urinary tract of mucus. The herbs comfrey, hyssop, fenugreek, thyme, and slippery elm together in capsules expel mucus from the digestive and respiratory tracts, and clear the sinuses. Avoid dairy products, chocolate, and fried foods, and smoking, as they will increase mucous secretion.

Mumps

Add three tablespoons of grated ginger root to a warm bath. Soak in this to rid the body of toxins. Soak a cloth in mullein tea and apply the cloth to the mumps to reduce swelling. Rub the spine with lobelia extract to help relax the spine. The herbs mullein and skullcap will help to heal and reduce swelling when taken orally. Take garlic and goldenseal in capsules to rid the body of infections and strengthen the natural defenses. Take lobelia and valerian to relax the system.

Nausea

To reduce upset stomach and vomiting take the following herbs as teas: red raspberry, ginger, peppermint, alfalfa, peach leaf, slippery elm, basil, or catnip. For relief of nausea chew ginger sticks or drink ginger tea. To prevent nausea take wild yam and vitamin B6 supplements.

Nerves

To heal the nervous system, prevent fatigue, eliminate hyperactivity, and calm emotions, take vitamin B6 and thiamine daily. Drink the following teas to relax the system and calm the nerves: chamomile, peppermint, spearmint, hops, catnip, horsetail, marshmallow or peach leaf. Drop primrose oil onto the tongue to calm nervous spasms.

Nightmares

Drink a tea made of hops or nettle to prevent night sweats. Take the herbs lobelia, skullcap, and yarrow in capsules to relax the mind before sleeping. Calcium, and vitamin D supplements, are helpful in the prevention of nightmares.

Nosebleed

Nosebleeds can be prevented by eating leafy green vegetables and by taking chlorophyll supplements. Both are rich in vitamin K. To reduce bleeding, take these herbs in combination: cayenne, goldenseal, or white oak bark.

Osteoporosis

Bone meal and dolomite contain calcium and magnesium. Take daily supplements to increase bone density. Animal protein causes calcium to be passed through the system through urination. Cut down on or eliminate the consumption of meat. Eat lots of green vegetables.

Pain

For quick relief, drink a strong tea made of St.-John's-wort, or lobelia, valerian, or cayenne extracts. Drink chamomile or peppermint tea for a mild sedative. Use the herbs valerian root, lobelia, cayenne, wild lettuce, or fenugreek to reduce pain and relax the system. Take vitamins E and C to reduce leg and calf pain.

Parasites

To prevent worms in kids and pets, drop a little black walnut extract into the mouth every few months for several days. Drink aloe vera juice to cleanse worms from the system. Many herbs have the ability to cleanse the body of worms. Some herbs are: garlic, taheebo, herbal pumpkin, cascara sagrada, papaya, bistort, sage, black walnut, chamomile, primrose root, and male fern. Eat pumpkin seeds and fresh garlic cloves to rid the body of parasites.

Pet Care

To clean a pet's system of worms, add papaya juice, black walnut extract, or garlic cloves to his diet for one week per month. Give your pet brewer's yeast or desiccated liver supplements to prevent fleas and produce a shiny, healthy coat. To rid a pet of tumors, add vitamin C to the diet.

Phlebitis

Apply vitamin E oil, or garlic oil to the affected area to reduce swelling and inflammation. Teas made from horseradish, chamomile, comfrey, pokeweed, or wintergreen also may be applied to aid in healing. Take the herbs goldenseal or garlic to reduce inflammation.

Take dolomite, and vitamins C and E to prevent blood clots, lessen pain, and speed healing.

Pituitary

Kelp, alfalfa, ginseng, gotu kola, yellow dock, parsley, and cayenne are herbs that will help to strengthen the pituitary gland. The herb lobelia will stimulate an under active pituitary while the herb licorice will lessen an overactive pituitary gland. Vitamins C and E work well with PABA and lecithin to normalize the pituitary.

Pleurisy

Make a rub using equal parts of lobelia, cayenne, and slippery elm tea. Mix them with cod liver oil and apply to the chest three to four times daily. Take the herb pleurisy root in capsules or as a tea to relax, heal, and reduce inflammation.

Poison Ivy

To stop itching and reduce blistering, apply one of the following to the skin: baking soda and water, aloe vera gel, lobelia extract, or jewelweed juice. Take the herb goldenseal and vitamin C daily to reduce inflammation. The herbs burdock and yellow dock will also promote healing when taken daily.

Poisoning

Immediately after poison is ingested, take activated charcoal to absorb poisons and pass them through the system. Take large doses of the herb lobelia to induce vomiting. To combat blood poisoning take the herbs chickweed, chamomile, or echinacea root. Eat two heads of iceberg lettuce to combat ptomaine poisoning.

Take vitamin A, C, and D along with folic acid to speed healing. See a doctor if a harmful toxin is ingested, or there is a drug overdose.

Polyps

Take vitamins C and E to clear up polyps and prevent lesions. To heal nose polyps mix equal parts of these powdered herbs: bayberry, bloodroot, and black pepper. Snuff the mixture up the nose frequently.

Pregnancy Tips

The herbs wild yam, red raspberry, false unicorn, and hawthorn will strengthen the uterus muscles, prevent miscarriage, and ward off cramps. Take cod liver oil, iodine, and iron to prevent morning sickness, and birth defects in your infant. Take dandelion, kelp, and alfalfa to provide minerals and keep weight off the hips. Alcohol consumption is the leading cause of birth defects and mental retardation in newborns and should be avoided at all stages of pregnancy. Smoking during pregnancy robs the baby of oxygen and contributes to colic.

Prickly Heat

Apply aloe vera gel, garlic oil, or cod liver oil to the affected area. Take vitamin A, C, D, and E, and zinc supplements to hasten recovery.

Prostate Gland

Parsley and juniper berries may be taken together to relieve a swollen prostate due to water retention. The herbs goldenseal and garlic fight infection in the prostate. The herb corn silk will fight painful urination due to prostate problems. The following hers prevent prostate problems: cayenne, ginger, ura ursi, and queen of the meadow. Bee pollen and ginseng together strengthen the prostate and promote physical endurance.

Psoriasis

Apply aloe vera gel, garlic oil, or an herbal tea of comfrey and goldenseal to the affected areas. Take cod liver oil, linseed oil, vitamin E, lecithin, and zinc to promote healing. The herbs chickweed, red clover, Redmond clay, yellow dock, and dandelion help when taken orally.

Rashes

Apply vitamin E oil; cod liver oil, or aloe vera gel, to the rash as often as needed. Take vitamins C and zinc to prevent rashes. Avoid the sun and hot water.

Rheumatism

Soak in a bath of warm water and rosemary to reduce pain and inflammation. Rub sore areas with garlic oil, lobelia, or an herbal tea of hops, comfrey, or horseradish. The following herbs may be taken in capsules to relieve inflammation and flush out deposits: parsley, alfalfa, and chaparral. Drink red raspberry tea to promote healing. The herb taheebo will help the body to resist the disease. The herbs willow and wintergreen can be taken like aspirin to relieve soreness. Take magnesium, calcium, and vitamins C and E to hasten the healing process.

Scarlet Fever

Use the powdered form of the herbs ginger or goldenseal to relieve pain and to open pores, so that

101

bacteria can be released. Add the herbs to a warm bath and soak. To relieve a sore throat, gargle with an herbal tea of bayberry. Drink red raspberry tea to hasten recovery. Use a catnip tea enema to release toxins from the body. Take the following herbs to let the body rest: lobelia, valerian root, yarrow, garlic, and cayenne.

Scars

Apply vitamin E oil, cod liver oil, or aloe vera gel, to wounds or burns to prevent scarring. Also apply the oils to scars to lessen coloration.

Senility

The following herbs will improve the memory, promote endurance and vitality, and retard the aging process: ginseng, gotu kola, dandelion, alfalfa, licorice, and yellow dock.

Shingles

Apply apple cider vinegar, peppermint oil, or an ointment of thyme and vitamin E oil, to the affected areas. Drink pennyroyal tea as often as possible. The herbs lobelia, valerian, bayberry, ginger, and cinnamon work well in healing shingles.

Shock

The herbs cayenne, lobelia, valerian, ginger, and myrrh may be used together or individually to decrease the symptoms of shock. Take vitamins C and E to speed recovery.

Skin Cracks

Apply the following as needed: aloe vera gel, black walnut extract, or Redmond clay. To soften tough skin cracks, take the herb don quai in capsules. Take extra zinc, and vitamins A, C, D, E, and B-complex.

Small Pox

Soak in a bath of warm water and grated ginger root. This will rid the body of infection. Drink an herbal tea of red raspberry, ginger, prickly ash, or cinnamon. Add a drop of lobelia or cayenne to the tea to relax the system. Take garlic tabs and fresh garlic cloves to ward off infection.

Smoking

Drink a tea made of the herbs lobelia, valerian, hops, chamomile, peppermint, and skullcap to lessen the desire for nicotine and calm the nerves. Drink catnip tea to lift the spirits. Take the herb echinacea in capsules to cleanse the lymphatic system that is often polluted by smoke.

Sore Throat/Tonsillitis

Place the following ingredients on a clean cloth: Garlic oil, lobelia extract, cayenne extract, warm salt water, and a tea made of comfrey or chickweed. Wear the cloth around the throat as often as possible. Marjoram tea with honey and lemon will soothe the throat and lessen coughing. Gargle with salt water, chlorophyll, or a tea of one of the following: red sage, eucalyptus, horehound, fenugreek, cayenne, lobelia, licorice, myrrh, bistort, yarrow, bayberry, witch hazel, peppermint, spearmint, or wintergreen. To help prevent sore throats, take juniper

103

berries in capsules. Drink aloe vera juice twice daily to soothe and heal the throat.

Snoring

Avoid sleeping on the back. Avoid eating and drinking before bed. Avoid fatty and salty foods.

Spleen Care

Take choline and vitamin C supplements to assist in the healing of an infected spleen. To prevent a swollen, inflamed spleen, the following herbs may be taken together or separately: horse radish, cascara sagrada, barberry, dandelion, yellow dock, cayenne, garlic, and ura ursi.

Sprains

Apply moist heat and ice alternately, to reduce pain, swelling, and inflammation. Rub the sore area with lobelia or cayenne extract or and herbal tea made of comfrey or marshmallow. Take lobelia or valerian root with cayenne to rest the body and allow healing.

Sterility

Take kelp, vitamin C, E, and B-complex to increase the chances of conception. The herb false unicorn helps to normalize the reproductive organs. The herb red clover may assist in restoring fertility. To increase sexual desire and to balance the hormones, the following herbs may be taken: ginseng, damiana, safflower, juniper, saw palmetto, chickweed, and plantain. To reduce sexual desire, the herbs hops, sage, and skullcap can be taken in capsules or teas.

104

Stiff Neck

Apply lobelia extract or mullein tea to the sore area and massage gently.

Sties

Apply cayenne extract or strawberry leaf tea to the sty to bring it to a head and to draw toxins from the area. Be careful when applying cayenne to the sty, because it will irritate the eye. Use a cotton swab to apply. Take lecithin, zinc, and cayenne and yellow dock. They will prevent sties from forming. Dandelion tea will cleanse the blood of bacteria that cause sty formation.

Stress

Drink "near-beer" a natural, non-alcoholic beverage made from hops, which will calm the entire system. When under stress, it is important to eat regularly, and to stick to a diet of whole foods, vegetables, and grains. Avoid caffeine, sugar, chocolate, and alcohol since these will only further tax the system. Take the herbs lobelia, valerian root, or hops in capsules or teas will relax the entire system. The herbs ginseng, cayenne, hawthorn, and gotu kola will provide energy and vitality.

Stretch Marks

Apply aloe vera gel, vitamin E oil, or cod liver oil to stretch marks to nourish and to heal them. To prevent stretch marks, eat plenty of nuts and seeds, and take zinc and vitamin A, C, D, E, and B-complex.

Sunburn

Always wear a moisturizing sunscreen when the skin is exposed to the sun. Avoid using baby oil or lotions that contain lanolin because they encourage as well as intensify burns. Apply aloe vera gel to the skin before and after sun exposure. Use a lotion that contains PABA to deepen a tan without excessive sun exposure. Apply chilled apple cider vinegar, aloe vera gel, or plantain frequently to a burn to nourish it. Try one of the following for a sun burnt face: Apply a mixture of milk and whole-wheat flour to the face. Leave until dry and remove with warm water. Rub olive oil onto a burnt face. Apply a paste of barley flour, honey, and raw egg white. Leave on for thirty minutes and then rinse with warm water.

Taste (loss of)

Zinc supplements help to improve the sense of taste. Take a daily mineral and vitamin supplement.

Thyroid Care

The following herbs will help to normalize thyroid activity: poke weed, Irish moss, kelp, parsley, and cayenne. The following herbs help heal an under active thyroid: bayberry, goldenseal, and myrrh.

Tooth Care

Brush the teeth with black walnut or strawberry leaf powder to remove plaque and restore enamel. The following herbs ease tooth pain, or a teething baby's painful gums: lobelia extract, cayenne extract, pennyroyal oil, oil of clove, or chamomile tea. Chewing on catnip leaves also eases pain. Take dolomite and bone meal

106

orally to strengthen teeth. Horsetail helps the body utilize calcium and thereby, strengthens tooth enamel. The herbs comfrey and alfalfa help prevent tooth decay. The herbs valerian root, wild lettuce, cayenne, and lobelia help to lessen a toothache. Take vitamin A, C, and D to ensure healthy teeth.

Ulcers

Avoid oily food, soda, sugar, and aspirin. They will only aggravate the ulcer further. Drink comfrey tea or liquid acidophilus culture frequently to soothe and to heal ulcers of the stomach and intestines. Ginger tea also acts as a natural antacid. To reduce internal bleeding of an ulcer, take chickweed and cayenne in capsules. The herbs comfrey, pectin, slippery elm, alfalfa, and horsetail help to coat the digestive tract and soothe stomach and colon ulcers. The following help to heal ulcers: bayberry, bistort, burdock, hops, hyssop, pennyroyal, pokeweed, sage, wild yam, yucca, red raspberry, myrrh, goldenseal, and white oak bark.

Varicose Veins

Apply vitamin E oil or a tea made of the following: comfrey, white oak bark, or witch hazel to the veins. The herbs white oak bark, bayberry, cayenne, and taheebo will help to heal as well as resist the disease. Cleanse the colon frequently. A full colon puts pressure on the arteries therefore exacerbating varicose veins.

Venereal Disease

See a doctor immediately. Always use latex condoms during anal, oral, or vaginal intercourse, to prevent the transmission of venereal disease or HIV.

Take the herb taheebo and garlic to fight infection. Douche with garlic and water twice daily to relieve inflammation and itching.

Vomiting

Sip an herbal tea made of peach bark, basil, or catnip, or sip honey water to settle your stomach. If there is blood in the vomit, see a doctor.

Warts

Apply cayenne extract, vitamin E oil, aloe vera gel, or a strong mandrake tea to the wart. Take the herbs buckthorn, red clover, chaparral, mandrake, or mullein in capsules to help rid the body of warts. Take niacin, PABA, and zinc to speed the elimination of warts.

Yeast Infection

Wear cotton panties. Cotton is a breathable natural fabric. Avoid nylon panty hose that contribute to the growth of yeast bacteria. Avoid brewer's yeast or any yeasty food that cause a yeast imbalance in the body. Douche with a tablespoon of garlic oil, acidophilus culture, or white vinegar in a pint of water. Take garlic and acidophilus supplements twice daily to hasten healing. Eat plain yogurt to rid the body of yeast infections. Plain yogurt may also be inserted directly into the vagina to relieve itch and inflammation. Eat plenty of fresh, raw garlic. A garlic clove may also be peeled and wrapped in cheesecloth and inserted into the vagina to speed healing. Remove after several hours.

Chapter 13: Natural Health Products Listing

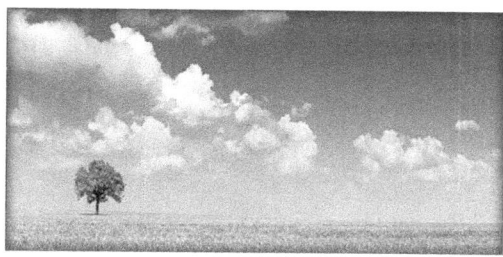

(The following natural health products are available in most health food stores)

A - Z

A

A-Retinyl Palmitate, Acerola, Acidophilus / Bifidus, Acne Control, Acne Relief, Aconitum Napellus, Adrenal, After Bath Powder, Alfalfa Leaf, Algae, All Greens, All-Purpose Seasoning, Allergies, Allergy Relief, Allergy Relief Tea, Allium Cepa, Aloe Vera, Aloe Vera Lotion / Gel / Juice, Alpha-Lipoic Acid, Amalaki (Indian Gooseberry), Amino Acids, Amyris, Anise Seed, Antacid, Anti-Aging / Wrinkle Creams, Anti-Oxidants, Antimonium Crudum, Antimonium Tartaricum, Apis Mellifica, Apple Cider Vinegar (Capsules), Apple Cider Vinegar (Liquid), ArabinoGalactan AG, Arnica Flower, Arnica Montana, Aromatherapy, Arsenicum Album,

Arthritic Pain, Artichoke, Ashwagandha, Asthma, Astragalus, Athlete's Ointment, Ayurvedic Herbs

B

Balsam Fir Needle, Barbecue Seasoning, Basil, Basil (Sweet), Bath Salts, Batteries, Bay, Bayberry, Bee Pollen, Belladonna, Bergamot, Beta-Carotene, Bilberry, Biochemic Phosphates, Bioflavonoids, Bioplasma, Biotin, Bismuth, Bitter Almond, Black Alder Bark, Black Catechu, Black Cohosh, Black Pepper, Black Tea, Black Walnut, Bladderwrack, Blessed Thistle, Blood Pressure, Blood Sugar, Bloodroot, Blue Cohosh, Bone Meal, Borage Oil, Boron-Silica, Boswellia, Bovine Colostrum, Breath Freshener, Brewers Yeast, Brigham Tea, Bromelain, Bryonia Alba, Bubble Bath, Buchu (African), bug bites and stings, Bugleweed, Bupleurum, Burdock Root, Butcher's Broom, Butea - Superba

C

Caffeine, Cajeput, Calcarea Flourica, Calcarea Phosphorica, Calcarea Sulphurica, Calcium, Calcium & Magnesium, Calcium Pangamate (B15), Calendula Flowers, California Poppy, Camphor, White, Candida Yeast, Cantharis, Caprylic Acid, Carbo Vegetabilis, Cardamon Seed, Carrot Seed, Cascara Sagrada, Cassia (Cinnamon), Castor Oil, Cat's Claw (Ulna de Gatos Vine), Cayenne, Cedarwood, Celandine, Celery Seed, Celestial Seasonings, Cellulite Control, Chamomile, Chamomile Tea, Chamomile, Wild, Chamomilla, Charcoal, Chickweed, Children's Remedies, Chitosan, Chlorella, Chlorophyll, Choline, Chondroitin Sulfate, Chromium, Chronic Fatigue Syndrome CFIDS, Cina (Wormseed), Cinnamon, Cinnamon Bark, Cinnamon Leaf, Cinnamon Spice, Circulatory System, CitriMax

(Weight Loss), Citronella, CLA - Conjugated Linoleic Acid, Clary Sage, Classic Herbal Blend Tea, Cleansing Pads, Cleansing Programs, Clove Bud, Cobalt, Cod Liver Oil, Coenzyme Q10 Reference, Coenzymes, Coffeacruda, Coffee Substitutes, Coleus Forskohlii, Collinsonia, Comfrey, Copper, Coriander Seed, Corn Silk, Corydalis Tubers, Cough & Cold, Cough & Cold Tea, Cough and Cold, Cramp Bark, Cranberry Juice Extract, Cranberry Tea, Creatine, Creatine Chews, Creatine Transport, Cyanocobalamin (B12), Cypress, Cysteine

D

D-Glutamate, D-Pantothenic Acid (B5), D-Ribose, Damiana, Dandelion, Desiccated Liver, Devil's Claw Extract, Devil's Club, Digestive Enzymes, Dish Detergent, Diuretic, DMAE, Dol-Mite, Dong Quai Extract.

E

Earache, Echinacea, Echinacea Tea, Eczema, Elderberry / Flower, Elecampane, Elemi, Elk Velvet Antler, Emu Oil, Energy Supplements, Essiac - Herbal Cancer Remedy, Eucalyptus, Eucalyptus (Lemon), Eucalyptus Oil, EVA - Elk Velvet Antler, Evening Primrose Oil, Eye Cream, Eyebright, Eyesight

F

Facial Toner, Fatigue, Fennel (Sweet), Fennel Seed, Fenugreek, Ferrum Phosphoricum, Feverfew, Fibre, Fir Needle, Fir Needle (Siberian), Flax Seed Oil, Flourine, Fo-Ti / He Shou Wu, Folic Acid, Foot Care, Frankincense, Fructose, Fruit Tea, Functional & Therapeutic Tea

G

Garlic, Garlic Herb Seasoning, Gaz Away, Gelsemium Sempervirens, Gentian Root, Geranium, Geranium (Bourbon), Geranium Root, Ginger, Ginger Root, Ginger Tea, Ginkgo Biloba, Ginseng, Ginseng Tea, GLA (Gamma Linolenic Acid), Glucosamine, Glucose Monitor, Glutamic Acid, Gold, Goldenseal, Gotu Kola, Grape Seed Extract, Grapefruit, Grapefruit Extract, Gravel Root, Green Cabbage, Green Tea, Green Tea Extract, Guarana, Guggulipid, Gymnema Sylvestre Extract

H

Hair and Scalp Care, Hair Inhibitor / Removal, Halibut Liver Oil, Hawthorn Berries, Hay Fever, Head Lice, Headache & Migraine, HeatherWorks Hair Loss, Helonias Root, Hemp Oil, Hepar Sulphuris Calcareum, Herbal Expectorant, herbest Complexion, HMB (Beta-Hydroxy BetaMethy.), Homeocoksinum, Hops Flowers, Horehound, Horse Chestnut, Horsetail, Household Cleaners, Hoxsey, Hypericum Perfoliatum, Hyssop

I

Ignatia Amara, Immortality Science, Inositol, Insect Bites and Stings, Insect Repellent, Insomnia, Insulin / Diabetes Supplies, Iodine, Ipeca (Ipecacuanha), Ipriflavone, Iron, Italian Seasoning

J

Jasmine, Juicing, Juniper Berries

K

112

Kali Muriaticum, Kali Phosphoricum, Kali Sulphuricum, Kava, Kava Kava Extract, Kelp (Fucus vesiculosus), Kidney, Kola Nut

L

L-Arginine, L-Glutamine, Lactase Enzyme, Lancing Devices, Laundry, Lavandin, Lavender, Lavender (Spike), Lavender Flowers, Laxative, Lecithin, Ledum Palustre, Leg Care, Lemon, Lemon Balm, Lemon Pepper Spice, LemonGrass, Licorice - DGL, Licorice Root, Ligustrum Berry, Lime, Lip Care, Lipoec, Liquid Aminos Seasoning, Liver Health, Lobelia, Lomatium, Lung Congestion, Lutein, Lycopene, Lycopodium Clavatum

M

Ma Huang, Magnesia Phosphorica, Magnesium, Magnets (Bio) & Water Magnets, Male Health, Malic Acid, Mandarin Orange, Manganese, Marjoram, Marjoram (Wild), Marshmallow Root, Massage & Body Oil, Maternity, Medical Reminders, Menopause, Menstruation Relief, Mental Alertness, Mercurius Vivus, Micellized Vitamins, Milagro Nail Care, Milk Thistle, Moducare / Multi-mune, Moisturizer, Motherwort, Mountain Ash (Fraxinus), MSM (MethylSulfonylMethane), Mugwort Leaf, Mullein Leaf/Flower, Multi-Vitamins / Minerals, Muscle Aches, Mushroom Extract, Myrrh, Myrtle

N

Natrum Muriaticum, Natrum Phosphoricum, Natrum Sulphuricum, Neroli, Nettle, Stinging, Niacinamide / Niacin (B3), Nickel, Nutmeg, Nux Vomica

O

Olive Leaf (Oleuropein), Orange (Sweet), Oregano, Oregano Leaf, Oregon GrapeRoot, Osha Root

P

P.M.S., Pain Relief, Palmarosa, Papain, Papaya Enzymes, Para Amino Benzoic Acid, Parasite Cleanse, Parsley, Passion Flower, Patchouli, Pau D'Arco Bark, Pectin, Peppermint, Peppermint Leaf, Peppermint Tea, Peru Balsam, Pet Shampoo, Petitgrain, Phosphatidyl Serine & PS-30, Phosphorus, Phosphorus. Pine, Plant Digest Enzymes, Plantain, Poppy Seed, Post-Workout Formula, Potassium, Power-Max Natural Steroids, Pregnancy / Fertility Test, Propolis, Prostate, Protein - Whey & Soy, PseudoEphedrine / Ephedrine, Psyllium, Pulsatilla, Pumpkin Seed Oil, Pumpkin Seeds, Pumpkorn, Pycnogenol French Pine Bark, Pygeum Bark, Pyridoxine (B6), Pyruvate (Energy/Weight Loss)

Q

Quassia Bark, Quercetin

R

Real Fruit, Red Clover, Red Raspberry Leaf, Red Rice Yeast, Red Root, Refreshers/Sprays, Reishi, Relaxing Tea, Rhubarb Root, Rhus Toxicodendron, Riboflavin (B2), RNA / DNA, Rose Hips, Rosemary, Rosewood, Rosewood Mirage, Royal Jelly, Ruta Graveolens, Rutin

S

Safflower, Sage, Sage Dalmation, Salmon Oil, SAM-e (S-adenosyl-methionine), Sandalwood, Sandalwood Mysore, Sarsaparilla Root, Sassafras, Savory, Saw Palmetto, Schizandra, Scudder's Alterative, Selenium, Senna Leaf, Sepia, Shampoo / Conditioner, Shark

Cartilage - Cancer, Shark Cartilage / Liver Oil, Shaving Oil, Sheep Sorrel, Shepherd's Purse, Silica, Silica. Silicea (Silica), Sinus, Skullcap, Sleep Aid, Sleep Tea, Slippery Elm Bark, Smoking Relief, Snoring Relief, Soaps, Natural, Soy Isoflavone, Soya Nuts, Spearmint, Spearmint Grove, Spirulina, Spongia Tosta, Spruce, Squaw Vine, St. John's Wort, Sterinols / Sterols, Stethoscope, Stevia, Stone Root, Stop Smoking! Stress, Stretch Mark Cream, Sugandh Kokila Bengal, Sulphur, Sulphur., Sun Damaged Skin, Sunflower Seeds, Swedish Bitters, Sweet Orange

T

Tabacum, Tagetes (Marigold), Tangerine, Tanning, Sunless Self Tanner, Tanning, Sunscreen / Sunblock, Tarragon, Taurine, Tea Tree Oil, Tea Tree Traditional, Teething, Thermometer, Thiamine (B1), Thuja Leaf / Occidentalis, Thyme, Thyme Greenwich, Thyme Leaf, Thyroid, Tofu, Tone-Max Cellulite Lotion, Toner, Toothpaste, Traditional Cleaning, Trail Mix, Tribulus Terrestris, Tumeric, Tuna Oil, Turmeric

U

Urea Cream, Usnea Lichen, Uva Ursi

V

Valerian Root, Valerian Root Oil, Vanadium, Vanilla, Vanilla Oil, Vanilla Tea, Vetiver, Vetiver Giraffe, Viagra Natural / Aphrodisiacs, Violet Leaf, Vitameal, Vitamin A, Vitamin B, Vitamin C, Vitamin D, Vitamin E, Vitamin E Cream /Therapy, Vitamins, Vitex Chasteberry

W

Weight / Bulk / Mass Gainers, Weight Control, Wheat Germ, White Willow, Wild Chamomile, Wild Cherry Bark, Wild Oats, Wild Yam, Willow Bark, Wintergreen, Wintergreen Gaultheria, Witch Hazel, Wormwood (Freesia)

Y

Yarrow, Yarrow Oil, Yellow Dock, Ylang Ylang, Yogurt, Yucca Root

Z

Zeaxanthin, Zinc

Chapter 14: Treatable Ailments Using Natural Protocols

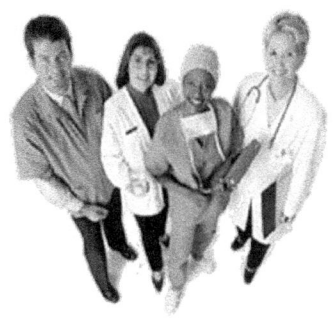

A - L

A

Abdominal Pain, Acid / Alkaline Balance, Acne, Acute Myocardial Insufficiency, Addison's Disease, Adrenal Glands, Aging, Alcoholism, Alimentary Canal, Alkylglycerols, Allergies, Alzheimer's Disease, Amenorrhea, Amoebas, Analgesia, Anaphylaxis, Anemia, Anesthesia, Angina, Anorexia Nervosa, Anti-bacterial, Anti-carcinogenic, Anti-edema, Anti-fungal, Anti-histamine, Anti-inflammatory, Anti-influenzal, Anti-microbial, Anti-tumor, Anti-yeast, Antibiotic, Antibodies, Antihepatotoxic, Antioxidants, Antipyretic, Antiseptic, Antispasmodic, Anxiolytic, Aphrodisiac, Appetite, Arrhythmias, Arteriosclerosis, Arthritis,

Asthma, Astringent, Ataxia, Arteriosclerosis (arteries hardening), Athlete's Foot, Atkins Diet, Attention Deficit Disorder (ADD)

B

Backache, Bacteria, Bad breath, Balance, Bedwetting, Bell's Palsy, Benign Prostatic Hyperplasia (BPH), Bile, Blackheads, Bladder irritations / infections, Bleeding Gums, Bleeding Piles, Blisters, Bloating, Blood Alliterative, Blood Cleanser, Blood Disorders, Blood Dyscrasias, Blood Glucose Levels, Blood Pressure, Blood Sugar Levels, Blood Toner, Bodybuilding / Athletic Performance, Boils, Bone Health, Bone Marrow, Bowel Problems / Inflammation, Brain Health, Breast Health, Breathing Problems, Broken Bone Support, Bronchial Muscles, Bronchitis, Brucellosis, Bruising, Burns, Bursitis/Tendonitis

C

Calcium Deficiencies, Calculi, Calluses, CAMP (Cyclic Adenosine Monophosphate), Cancer, Canker sores, Capillaries, Carbohydrate Metabolism, Carbuncles, Cardiac Weakness, Cardiovascular system, Carminative, Carpal Tunnel Syndrome, Catabolic Wastes, Cataracts, Catarrh, Cellular Health, Cellulite, Cervical Health, Chemical Sensitivity, Chemotherapy Support, Chicken Pox, Chilblains, Chlamydia spp., Choleretic, Cholesterol, Chronic Fatigue Syndrome (CFS), Circulation Problems, Cirrhosis, Clarity, Clean Water, Coagulation of Blood, Cold Sores, Colds and Chills, Colic, Colitis, Collagen Deficient Disorders, Colon Disease, Complexion, Confusion, Congealed Blood, Congestion, Congestive Heart Failure, Conjunctivitis, Connective Tissue Support, Constipation, Contractions, Convulsions, Corpus

118

Luteum, Coryza, Coughs, Cramps, Croup, Cuts and abrasions, minor, Cystitis, Cysts

D

Dandruff, Decongestant, Deficient Constitutions, Degenerative Disorders, Dementia, Demulcent, Dental Support, Deodorizer, Depression, Depurative, Dermatitis, Dermatological Conditions, Detox / Toxicity, Diabetes, Diabetic Neuropathy of the Foot, Diaper Rash, Diaphoretic, Diarrhea, Diet, Digestion, Disney, Diuretic, Diverticulitis, Dizziness (Vertigo), DNA / RNA, Dropsy, Dry Skin, Duodenal Ulcer, Dysmenorrhea, Dyspepsia, Dysplasia

E

E. Coli. Earache, Eczema, Edema, Emollient, Emotional Health, Emphysema, Endocrine System, Endometriosis, Energy, Enteric Bacterial Imbalance, Enteritis, Enuresis, Environmental Factors, Environmentally Safe, Enzyme Adenylate Cyclase, Enzymes, Epilepsy, Epstein-Barr Virus (EBV), Essential Fatty Acid Deficiency, Estrogen Production / Metabolism, Exhaustion, Expectorant, Eye and ear infection, Eyesight failing

F

False Labor, Fatigue, Fertility, Fever, Fibromyalgia, Fibrositis, First-Aid, Flatulence, Flu, Food Allergies, Food Poisoning, Food Sensitivities, Foot Care, Free Radicals, Fungal Infections.

G

Gallbladder, Gallstones, Gas, Gastric Juices, Gastro-Enteritis, Gastrointestinal Tract, General pain and healing, Genitourinary System Infections, Geriatrics,

Germicidal Disinfectant, Giardia, Gingivitis, Glandular Fever, Glaucoma, Globulin, Glucose Metabolism, Glycogen, Goiter, Gout,

H

Hair loss, Hair removal, Hair retardant, Hay Fever, Head Lice, Headache / migraine, Healthy skin - hair - nails, Hearing Loss, Heart Problems, Heartburn, Hemorrhages, Hemorrhoids, Hepatitis, Hepatotoxic Agents, Hernia, Herpes Simplex, High triglycerides, Hives, Hormones, Hot flashes, Hyperactivity, Hyperglycemia, Hypersensitivity, Hypertension (High Blood Pressure), Hypochloridia, Hypoglycemia, Hypokalemia, Hypotension, Hypoxia, Hysteria

I

Imbalance, General Systematic, Immunity, Impotence, Incontinence, Indigestion, Infant (5 - 12 Months), Infections, Inflammation, Injuries, Insect Bites and Bee Stings, Insomnia - restlessness, Insulin, Intestinal Disorders, Iron Deficiency, Irritability, Irritated / Itchy skin, Ischemic Heart Disease

J

Jaundice, Joint Pain / Health

K

Kidney

L

Labor Support / Promotion, Lactose Intolerance, Laryngitis, Laxative, Leg Pain, Leg Ulcers, Leukocyte / Macrophage Activity, Leucorrhoea, Lice, Liver,

Longevity, Lumbar Pain, Lung Health, Lupus, Lymph Node, Lymphatic Infections

M - Y

M

Macular Degeneration, Meal Replacement, Measles, Memory - brain / cognitive abilities, Menopause symptoms, Menorrhagia, Menses, Menstruation Problems, Mental Health, Metabolism, Metrorrhagia, Micturition, Milk Production, Mitral Valve Prolapse, Monoamine Oxidase, Mononucleosis, Moodiness, Morning Sickness, Motion Sickness, Mouth / Throat Inflammation, Mouth Ulcers, Mucous Membranes, Mumps / measles / small pox, Muscle Mass, Muscle Relaxant, Muscle Strain, Muscle Twitch, Musculature, Myocardial Degeneration

N

Nasal Infections, Nausea / abdominal cramps, Nephritis, Nerve Health / Pain, Nervine, Nervousness / Nervous System, Neuralgia, Neurological Pain, Night-Time Vision, Nocturnal Emission, Nose Bleeds, Nursing Mothers, Nutrition / Good Health

O

Osteoarthritis, Osteomalacia, Osteoporosis, Ovarian Health, Ovulation, Oxygenation

P

Pain, Palpitations, Panacea (All Healing), Pancreas, Parasitic Infections, Parkinson's Disease, Pelvic Atony, Pelvic Inflammatory Disease, Pelvic Viscera, Peptic Ulceration, Pernicious Anemia, Perspiration, Petit Mal,

Phlebitis, Phlegm, Photosensitivity, Physical Endurance, Pigmentation, Pituitary Gland, Pleurisy, PMS, Poison Ivy, Postpartum Depression, Potassium-Deficiency, Prebiotic, Pregnancy, Prolapse Syndromes, Prostate, Prostatitis, Protein, Psoriasis, Pus Discharge, Pyelitis

R

Rashes, Raynaud's disease, Rectal Engorgement, Red Blood Cells, Reflexes, Rehabilitation, Relaxant, Renal Excretions / Health, Reproductive System, Resistance, Respiratory Problems, Restless Legs Syndrome, Restlessness, Retro-Virus, Rheumatism, Rheumatoid Arthritis, Rheumatoid Neuralgia, Rickets, Ringworm, Rough, damaged skin

S

Saliva, Salmonella, Sanitizer, Scabies, Scaly Skin, Scars, Sciatica, Scurvy, Seborrhea, Sedative, Sedimentation, Seizures, Senility, Sensitive skin, Serenity, Serous Otitis Media (Fluid in the Ear), Sesame Street, Sex Hormone Production, Sexual Dysfunction, Shaking, Shaving, Shingles (Herpes zoster), Sinus Infection, Skin Disorders, Skin Ulcers, Sleep, Smoking, Snoring, Soothing, Sore Throat, Spasmolytic, Speech difficulty, Spermatorrhea, Spinal Concerns, Spleen, Sprains, Stamina, Staph. Spp., Sterility, Steroids - Natural, Stiffness, Stomach Problems, Strength, Strep. Spp., Stress / anxiety, Stretch Marks, Stroke, Sugar Metabolism, Sunburn, Sweetener, Swelling

T

Tachycardia, Tanning, Teeth and gum problems, Teething, Tendonitis, Tension, Throat Infections, Thrombocytes, Thymus Gland, Thyroid, Tinnitus ("ringing in the ears"), Tissue Health / Elasticity, Tonic,

Tonsillitis, Toxemia, Trachea, Trauma, Travel Sickness, Tremors, Trichomonas, Triglycerides, Tuberculosis, Tumors

U

Ulcers, Ultraviolet Radiation, Urethritis, Urinary Tract System, Urticaria, Uterine Atony, Uterine Bleeding, Uterine Fibroids, Uterine Pains

V

Vaginal infection, Varicose Veins, Varicosities, Vascular Conditions, Vasodilator, Vata Constitution, Vein Health, Vertigo, Viral Conditions, Visual Acuity, Visual Problems / Fatigue, Vitality, Vitiligo, Vomiting

W

Warts, Waste Excretion, Water Retention, Weakness, Weight Gain, Weight Loss / Obesity, Well-being, White Blood Cells, Whooping Cough, Womb Health, Worms, Ringworms, Tapeworms, Wounds and Skin Conditions, Wrinkles

Y

Yeast Infection - Candida Albicans

Chapter 15: Male/Female Sexuality

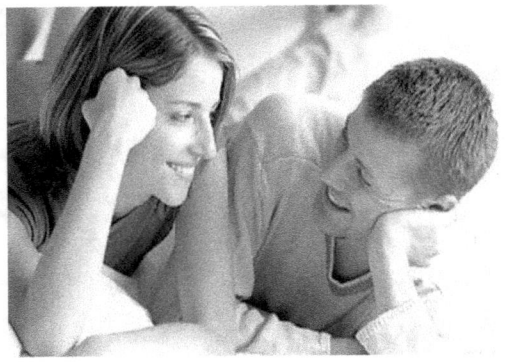

All sex hormones are made from cholesterol. Cholesterol is highly dependent on chromium for the correct synthesis of it. Since chromium body-stores decrease with age, it is important to replace chromium on a daily basis. In males, the organ most affected by chromium reduction, due to aging, are the testes.

The male sex gland, the testes, is responsible for the production of sperm and the secretion of testosterone. Testosterone, the hormone responsible for male sexual desire, is dependent on Vitamin E to produce sperm and to provide strong masculine features. Zinc is also a mandatory sex hormone nutrient.

124

Sperm contains calcium, magnesium, and zinc, and calcium deficiencies are evidenced in men who experience pre-mature ejaculation.

Nutrients required to be present in sufficient quantities for men to perform sex are:

1. Vitamin E ~ for testosterone

2. Zinc Monomethionine ~ for sperm counts

3. Chromium Polynicotinate ~ for sex hormones made from cholesterol

4. Boron ~ reduces the loss of calcium

5. Calcium ~ sperm = calcium, magnesium, and zinc

6. Magnesium ~ for sperm count

7. Niacin

The female sex glands, the ovaries, are responsible for the production of estrogen and progesterone. In order for these two female hormones to function properly, they require Vitamin E and niacin. These nutrients are vital components in maintaining female hormone function. For women taking birth control pills, vitamin deficiencies are common. Birth control pills destroy Vitamin E and several of the B-complex vitamins. Estrogen, found in birth control pills, and inorganic iron, are the major antagonists to Vitamin E. Birth control pills also interfere with fat metabolism. Most women experience bloating as a result of water retention. Excess water (edema) is uncomfortable as well as causes irritability due to sodium retention. Potassium alleviates both of these problems.

Nutrients required to be present in sufficient quantities for women to perform sex are:

    1. Vitamin E ~ for estrogen and progesterone production

    2. Chromium Polynicotinate ~ for sex hormones made from cholesterol

    3. Potassium ~ regulates water balance

    4. Niacin ~ for estrogen and progesterone production

    5. Boron

Sexual Dysfunction & Paraphilias:

    * Sexual problems are divided into different categories: *sexual dysfunctions* and *paraphilias*.

    * Sexual Dysfunctions pertain to one's ability to *perform* in a sexual capacity.

    * Paraphilias on the other hand, pertain to the stimuli the person needs in order that they become aroused.

    * There are nine sexual dysfunctions listed in the *DSM-IV* (the manual all mental health professionals use as a diagnostic guideline), four of which represent the male and the female version of a similar affliction. For example,

    * "Male Erectile Disorder" (impotence) and "Female Sexual Arousal Disorder" both describe a failure of the arousal system due to psychological/emotional reasons.

126

* "Male Orgasmic Disorder," and "Female Orgasmic Disorder." Not surprisingly, these refer to either a delay, or a complete absence, of orgasm following normal sexual arousal and stimulation.

* "Hypoactive Sexual Desire Disorder" (i.e., lack of sexual desire), and "Sexual Aversion Disorder" (extreme aversion and/or avoidance of sexual activity).

* "Premature Ejaculation Disorder," (self-explanatory), "Dyspareunia" (pain during intercourse), and "Vaginismus" (the muscles of the vagina contract, making penetration difficult or impossible).

* Nutritional deficiencies are the leading cause of most sexual dysfunction.

* The leading nutritional deficiency is chromium. Chromium's main function in the body is to activate insulin.

* Sperm contains the highest concentration of calories than any other body fluid.

* Blood contains the most nutrients than any other body fluid.

Appendix #1: Body System Charts

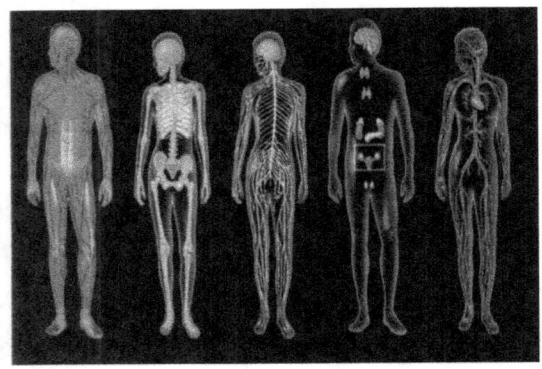

Please be advised that I have to make a legal disclaimer now: I do not endorse/ recommend, suggest or promote any of the products, devices, and or protocols on any of the pages contained herein. Nor do I suggest that you avoid a medical practitioner for any reason. I make no claim whether implied or written

The Endocrine System

Pineal

The function of the Pineal is not well understood; this gland has been referred to as the "third eye." Its only

128

major secretion is melatonin, which influences sleep cycles. It is strongly influenced by cycles of daylight, and is found in the limbric part of the brain.

Hypothalamus

The Hypothalamus is not a true endocrine gland; the hypothalamus is the main control center for virtually all organs and tissues. It regulates involuntary nervous system activity (flight or fight responses) and governs most physical expressions of emotions. It is critical for regulating overall homeostasis, including sleep cycles, food intake, body temperature, and thirst. It controls hormone production of the pituitary gland, which in turn, stimulates other endocrine glands to release hormones; therefore, the hypothalamus influences the entire endocrine network. It is also found in the limbic brain.

Parathyroid

The Parathyroid is critical for regulating blood calcium levels (which itself is critical for homeostasis) by pulling calcium from the bones and reabsorbing it through the kidneys. It also contributes to phosphorus and vitamin D metabolism. It is on the thyroid gland.

Pituitary

The Pituitary, about the size of a pea, is considered the "master gland" because many of its secretions regulate hormone production in the other endocrine glands. Its own hormones affect cell growth, protein synthesis, glucose utilization, fat metabolism, and the regulation of most chemical reactions in general. Found in the limbic brain.

Thyroid

The Thyroid is the body's major regulator of metabolic activity, primarily through the oxidation of glucose and oxygen consumption. It helps regulate food and calcium metabolism, body temperature, tissue, bone and nervous system development, and is essential for the development and regulation of the female reproductive system. It also affects protein synthesis, heart function, blood pressure and respiration. It is found in the neck.

Adrenal

The Adrenal is found on top of the kidneys, the adrenals function as two separate glands. They utilize cholesterol to synthesize dozens of steroid hormones that help regulate fluid electrolyte balances (especially sodium), affect sex drive, stimulate the body into "flight or fight" action, and at the same time maintain a state of "crisis management". In terms of sheer stress response, the adrenal glands are the star players.

Thymus

The Thymus is considered essential for the normal development of the immune response. It activates lymphocytes to recognize specific pathogens. It is located behind the breast bone.

Ovary

The Ovary produces estrogens and progesterone, which affect all aspects of the development of sexual activity. They also help regulate cholesterol levels and calcium.

Testes

The testes are a gland that produces the male reproductive cells and the male hormone testosterone.

Prostaglandin

Prostaglandin is considered to be "local" hormones, found in virtually all cell membranes. There many functions include hormone regulation, gastric secretion, platelet aggregation, and inflammation responses.

Uterus

The uterus contains and nourishes the embryo and fetus, and aids in balancing hormones.

Prostate

The prostate is partly glandular and partly muscular. The gland secretes a thin opalescent, slightly alkaline fluid that forms part of the semen.

The Digestive System

The digestive system is much more than just a place to put the things we eat. It is a complex refinery that converts foodstuffs into the majority of the nutritional tools we need to maintain health and wellness. If these are not viable options – if any part of the food processing operation becomes compromised through injury, substance abuse, or poor dietary habits – then the digestive system becomes a pathway to potential toxicity.

Parotid Gland

The Parotid Gland is a large salivary gland near the ear, stimulated to produce saliva by the presence of food in the mouth. Saliva contains certain antibodies and enzymes that play a major role in preventing pathogens from entering the body.

Temporomandibular Joint

The Temporomandibular Joint facilitates chewing, which, with the stimulation of saliva mixed with food, is the most significant process in the prevention of absorbing parasites.

Stomach Acid

Stomach Acid contains hydrochloric acid, which not only is a significant pathogenic inhibitor; it is also required to activate the stomach enzyme pepsin, which begins the breakdown of proteins for further processing in the small intestine. Without pepsin, proteins can begin to putrefy in the stomach.

Gallbladder

The Gallbladder is a "way" station for liver bile and can accumulate toxins, especially those of synthetic chemical origins.

Intrinsic Factor

Intrinsic Factor is produced only n the stomach and is a substance required for the absorption of B-12 in the small intestine.

Liver

The Liver is the primary site for the enzymatic breakdown of toxins and their subsequent removal via the kidneys and intestines.

Pancreas

The Pancreas produces most of the protease, lipase, and amylase (all digestive enzymes) involved in digestion, as well as juices that neutralize stomach acid in the small intestine.

Small Intestine

The Small Intestine is the recipient of all foods and digestive juices and its function can be affected by any imbalances in the stomach, pancreas, liver and / or gallbladder.

Valve Houston

The Valve Houston is one of the mucosal folds of the rectum, and plays a role in controlling intestinal parasites.

Large Intestines

The Large Intestines reabsorb water from undigested materials and eliminates the consolidated waste. The "friendly" bacteria of the gut provide some digestion, but mostly contribute to controlling the growth and spread of harmful bacteria, and to the production of some B-complex vitamins and vitamin K.

Bowl Flora

Bowl Flora provides the best defense against invading harmful bacteria in the gut.

Ileocecal Valve

The Ileocecal Valve prevents fecal material from backing up into the small intestine.

Micelle Balance

Micelles are micro-clusters of fat-based molecules that transport nutrients through the small intestine. Bioenergetically, micelle balance represents the body's capacity to absorb and regulate the distribution of nutrients.

The Immune System

Detoxification itself is a defensive measure, but it is assisted greatly by the immune system proper. The immune system might be considered the border guard of our protective network. A healthy immune system is critical to the balanced body. This does not mean an immune system that is constantly stimulated, but rather one that is fully functional, conserving its resources and ready to do battle when necessary. "Necessary" results from injury, invasion or imbalance. The first two are usually temporary responses, but the imbalance can trigger the immune system for the long haul.

Lymphatic

The Lymphatic System is our first line of internal defense; a vast network of drainage ducts and glands designed to remove wastes, toxins and pathogens from the blood via a plasma-like fluid called lymph. The lymphatic network is also critical to supporting the cardiovascular system by returning leaked fluids to the bloodstream.

Brain

Our thought processes have direct impacts on the chemicals released by the brain, which in turn stimulate the autonomic (involuntary) nervous system to respond to incoming and perceived stressors.

Thymus

The Thymus produces specific lymphocytes to attack viruses, bacteria and abnormal cell growths.

Tonsils / Adenoids

The Tonsils / Adenoids are sites of concentrated lymph tissue for trapping and destroying bacteria entering the body through ingestion or inhalation.

Liver

The Liver is the primary site for the enzymatic breakdown of toxins and their subsequent removal via the kidneys and intestines.

Skin

The Skin is the largest detoxifying organ of the body, and is capable of exerting as many toxins as the kidneys through its oil glands and sweat pores. The Skin is our first line of external defense.

Appendix

The Appendix is a major lymphoid organ, ideally situated for processing the bacteria of the large intestine.

Bowl Flora

Bowl Flora provides the best defense against invading harmful bacteria in the gut.

Bone Marrow

Bone Marrow is the site of red blood cell and lymphocyte (white blood cell) production.

Connective Tissue

135

Connective Tissue is the most abundant and widespread tissue in the body. Home to the meridian system, it is the primary communication network of the body in terms of the bionetic information that serves to maintain homeostasis and health. It becomes the depository for many of the toxins that are not completely metabolized or eliminated through the normal processes of detoxification.

The Lymphatic System

The massive network of the lymphatic system is our first line of internal defense. Twice as extensive as the circulatory system, it removes pathogens and waste products from the bloodstream and sends them through a series of vessels that occasionally expand into areas of concentrated lymphoid tissue called "node", where the pathogens are destroyed by lymphocytes and macrophages. The cleansed lymph is then returned to the bloodstream through the subclavian veins. The fluid known as "lymph" does not move actively through the system, but relies on the physical action of the skeletal muscles and diaphragm for transport. Even so, the lymph movement is slow and uneven, emphasizing the grave importance of physical activity in maintaining overall health. Another critical factor to health is the lymph's role in returning interstitial and plasma proteins to the bloodstream. This fluid is forced out of the blood when it moves from the arterial capillaries to venous capillaries. Although the amount is relatively small – about three liters per day – this fluid must be returned to the bloodstream for the cardiovascular system to function properly. Thus, if the lymphatic is to serve us, we must serve the lymph! Since the function of the various lymph vessels is basically the same, we will describe here only the areas of drainage.

Subclavian (Trunks)

The Subclavian Trunks drains the upper arms.

Cervical (Nodes)

Cervical Nodes are located near the cervical vertebrae, servicing the head and trunk.

Lymphoreticular (Tissue)

Lymphoreticular Tissue is pertaining to the mesh-like network of cells that forms the lining of the lymphatic vessels.

Axillary (Nodes)

Axillary Nodes are found in the chest near the armpits.

Right Nymphatic (Duct)

The Right Nymphatic Duct drains the right arm and the right side of the head and thorax.

Thoracic (Duct)

The Thoracic Duct drains the rest of the body.

Abdominal (Nodes)

The Abdominal Nodes are found throughout the abdomen, but mainly clustered around the abdominal aorta.

Cysterna Chyli

The Cysterna Chyli is an enlarged sac of the thoracic duct that collects lymph from the legs and abdomen.

Inguinal (Nodes)

The Inguinal Nodes are located in the groin area.

Peripheral (Nodes)

The Peripheral Nodes are scattered throughout the connective tissue in the outlying areas of the body.

I Have a Special Gift for My Readers

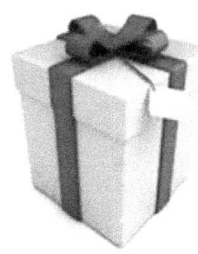

I appreciate my readers for without them I am just another author attempting to make a difference. If my book has made a favorable impression please leave me an honest review. Thank you in advance for you participation.

My readers and I have in common a passion for the written word as well as the desire to learn and grow from books.

My special offer to you is a massive ebook library that I have compiled over the years. It contains hundreds of fiction and non-fiction ebooks in Adobe Acrobat PDF format as well as the Greek classics and old literary classics too.

In fact, this library is so massive to completely download the entire library will require over 5 GBs open on your desktop.

Use the link below and scan all of the ebooks in the library. You can select the ebooks you want individually or download the entire library.

The link below does not expire after a given time period so you are free to return for more books rather than clog your desktop. And feel free to give the link to your friends who enjoy reading too.

I thank you for reading my book and hope if you are pleased that you will leave me an honest review so that I can improve my work and or write books that appeal to your interests.

Okay, here is the link…

http://tinyurl.com/special-readers-promo

PS: If you wish to reach me personally for any reason you may simply write to mailto:support@epubwealth.com.

I answer all of my emails so rest assured I will respond.

Meet the Author

Dr. Harry Jay is Director of Research for AppliedMindSciences.com, a mental health and mind research group of Applied Web Info, and is the author of over 100 books and research papers as a behavioral scientist.

In his 32-year career, Dr. Harry Jay has contributed many new mental health treatment treatments and protocols using some of the new advances he has discovered in Energy Psychology.

He specializes in addictions of all kinds, sexual abuse, child predation and gender relationships.

He is also a board member to ePubWealth.com and serves on the science committee assisting non-fiction science writers in book publishing and promotion.

As a leading behavioral scientist, he provides profiling services to the company's ForensicsNation.com unit as well as criminal psychology research to aid in identifying and apprehending child predators and cyber-criminals of all kinds.

He resides in Southern Utah and enjoys the outdoors, fishing and photography.

141

http://www.amazon.com/author/harryjay

Visit some of his websites
http://www.AddMeInNow.com
http://www.AppliedMindSciences.com
http://www.AppliedWebInfo.com
http://www.BookbuilderPLUS.com
http://www.BookJumping.com
http://www.EmailNations.com
http://www.EmbarrassingProblemsFix.com
http://www.ePubWealth.com
http://www.ForensicsNation.com
http://www.ForensicsNationStore.com
http://www.FreebiesNation.com
http://www.HealthFitnessWellnessNation.com
http://www.Neternatives.com
http://www.PrivacyNations.com
http://www.RetireWithoutMoney.org
http://www.SurvivalNations.com
http://www.TheBentonKitchen.com
http://www.Theolegions.org
http://www.VideoBookbuilder.com

**Some Other Books You May Enjoy From
ePubWealth.com, LLC Library Catalog**

EPW Library Catalog Online
http://www.epubwealth.com/wp-
content/uploads/2013/07/Leland-benton-private-turbo.pdf

EPW Library Catalog Download
http://www.filefactory.com/f/562ef3ea1a054f0a

www.ingramcontent.com/pod-product-compliance
Lightning Source LLC
Chambersburg PA
CBHW070115290526
45789CB00005B/2030